More from The Maui Vegetarian

He's back again! Chef Brian creates more
unique and mouth-watering recipes designed to
enhance your health program, and all in good
taste. Browse through the photos of these
delicious, kitchen-tested (and kid-tested!)
dishes that will take you to a place words can't
describe. Included in this sequel to
The Maui Vegetarian...Cooking with Aloha,
you will find additional facts about food as well
as more tips from Chef Brian on how you can
make food preparation simple and tasteful.
Our hope is that you will be inspired to
experiment in your own kitchen, even using
creative presentations, and never cease to
learn. The sky's the limit.   Keep on that *tasty*
road to good health where you will reap the
benefits of energy, life, and clearness of mind.
Our prayer and hope for you is that the Lord
who made the heaven and the earth and all
that's in it, including YOU, will bless you
abundantly in every facet of your life,
for His glory and honor.
May you be blessed by what is presented here.
With love in Christ our Lord and Savior,
Aloha...The Maui Vegetarian

Printed by Sunquest Inc. Shanghai, China
Published and created by Brian Igarta
Copyrighting © in January 2010 Library of Congress

This book is dedicated to my Dad, Buddy & Mom, Diana, from whom I inherited the diversity of my nationality and my Hawaiian roots. Thank you for all that you taught me and for putting up with me all those times I drove you crazy. Through it all you still called me son.

JOB 1:21 and said, Naked came I out of my mother's womb, and naked shall I return thither: the LORD gave, and the LORD hath taken away; blessed be the name of the Lord.

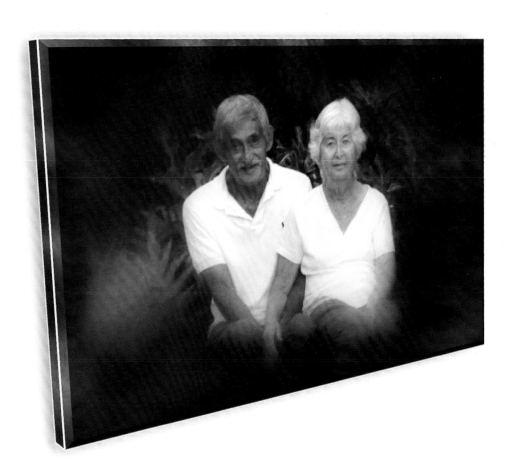

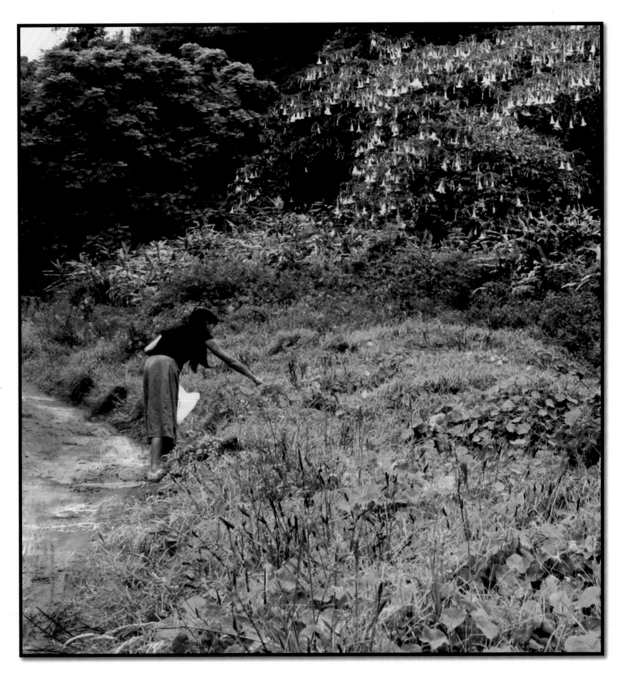

Nasturtium leaves are used as a tea to treat coughs, colds and the flu, as well as menstrual and respiratory difficulties. High in vitamin C, nasturtiums also act as a natural antibiotic and were used topically as a poultice for minor cuts and scratches. Here, my wife picks a bag full of fresh nasturtium flowers to add color and flavor to our green salads.

Contents

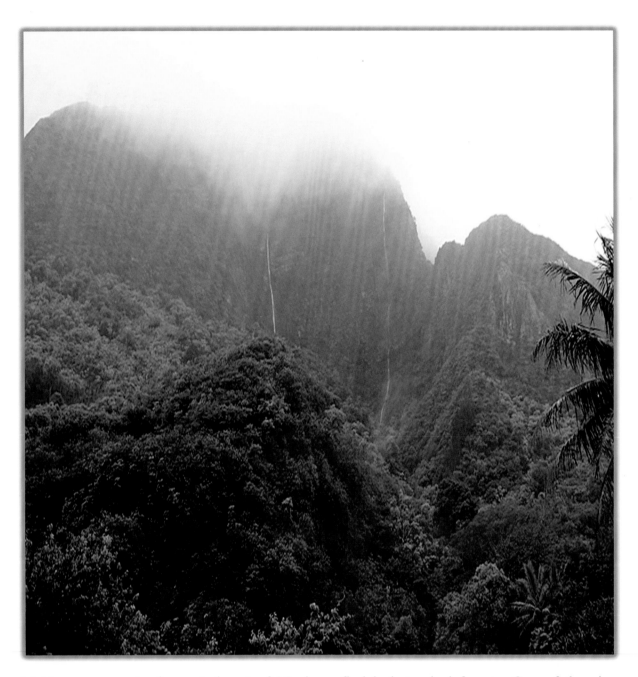

Making our way to the central part of Maui we find lush tropical forest. One of the nice amenities of living on an island like this is that nature is your refrigerator. This place is great for foraging fresh, natural foods. We can find Hawaiian ginger root, guava, passion fruit, coconut, bananas, berries and many other kinds of edibles as well as traditional Hawaiian medicinal plants for healing.

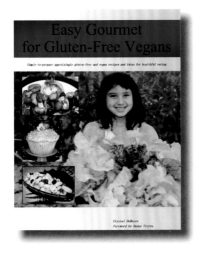 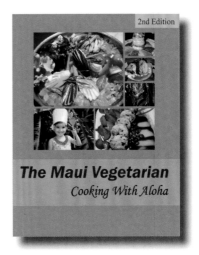

For more wonderful recipes, and other useful information, try another of our books created with a healthful lifestyle in mind. Please feel free to send your comments and concerns to our web site.

www.TheMauiVegetarian.com

By John Westerdahl, PhD, MPH, RD, CNS

"You are what you eat" and modern medical science has well established that what you eat has a major effect on your health and wellness. Yes, "what you eat today is walking and talking tomorrow." The nutrients found in the foods you eat eventually become a part of your body. This is why it is essential to put the healthiest and most natural whole foods possible into your body. Live foods (fruits, vegetables, whole grains, legumes, healthy herbs, nuts, seeds and other healthy plant foods) produce live, healthy bodies. Dead foods (meats, poultry, fish and the dead flesh of other animals and their byproducts, dairy products, eggs, refined and overly processed foods including sugar and refined grains products, hydrogenated and trans fats, unhealthy chemical food additives and preservatives, chemically created foods, etc.) lead to illness, disease and death. Today's health science research has confirmed that populations who eat plant-based or vegetarian diets enjoy better health and age more slowly compared to their heavy meat-eating counterparts. There are many reasons why vegetarian diets play a critical role in preventing disease and are key to achieving optimal health and longevity. Studies show the vegetarian diets are optimal for preventing, controlling and even reversing diseases such as heart disease and Type-2 Diabetes. This is because healthy vegetarian diets tend to be very low in saturated fat and cholesterol, while high in fiber and heart-protective compounds found in plants. There is strong scientific evidence that a diet rich in fruits and vegetables protect us against many forms of cancer. Many scientists believe that the natural phytochemicals found in plant foods like carotenoids, vitamin C and E, selenium, indoles, isothiocyanates, flavonoids, phenols, limonene and others are the powerful protective anti- cancer compounds. Many of the protective compounds also prevent against stroke and other diseases and illnesses as well. We need to include more plant foods in our diets every day. Nutritional science continues to discover that plant foods are powerful healing foods. In determining the best diet to optimize the healing powers of plant foods, adhering to a healthy whole foods vegan vegetarian diet is the optimal way to go for health, wellness, disease prevention and treatment, anti-aging and longevity.

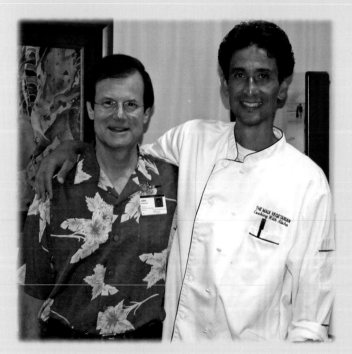

A healthy vegan vegetarian diet is powerful medicine! For the past several years I have had the privilege of being a good friend and colleague of Chef Brian Igarta. I have worked with Brian from planning and presenting community-based vegetarian cooking classes to conducting vegetarian cuisine cooking demonstrations to physicians, registered dietitians and other health professionals. My family and I have personally prepared and enjoyed many of his excellent vegetarian recipes in our home kitchen. Chef Igarta is a culinary master at creating wonderful and delicious health promoting recipes. His first cookbook, *The Maui Vegetarian* was a well-received contribution to the field of vegetarian cuisine. In his new book, *The Maui Vegetarian-Hana Hou*, Brian has created more wonderful recipes that you and your family will enjoy. In this new book, Brian at the request of many of his fans and friends who live busy lifestyles, has created many "quick and easy" recipes that can easily be prepared in little time. I encourage you to try all the recipes in this cookbook. You will experience a delightful new adventure in healthy eating.

John Westerdahl, PhD, MPH, RD, CNS is a nutritionist, registered dietitian, master herbalist, Board Certified Anti-Aging Health Practitioner, health educator and health scientist. Dr. Westerdahl is an internationally recognized expert in the fields of nutrition, wellness and Lifestyle Medicine.

Our nation is experiencing skyrocketing rates of obesity and diabetes in adults and even in children. Every family and individual needs to take a good look at what they are eating. The Standard American Diet, which is the typical diet, is loaded with sugar, refined white products, and animal fats. Let's stop sacrificing ourselves and our children to the food gods and go back to the Edenic Diet (the original diet in the Garden of Eden as God intended) as much as possible. Through education, good diet practices, and staying away from harmful foods and habits, it's possible to change how we feel, think and act for the better. Start by taking small steps, understanding that you will pay now or pay later down the road, so be willing to make some sacrifices. Medical, scientific, and Biblical studies show that we can have a better quality of life when we choose to fuel our bodies with the right food sources. There is so much information out there to prevent us from suffering needless ailments and death, there is no excuse. Most of the illnesses and diseases people suffer from come from diet and lifestyle habits, we can change hereditary factors to be positive and thus, pass on good health and habits to the generations after us. Start now by educating yourself and doing the best you can, then leave the rest to the Creator. Choose certified organic as much as possible, eating lots of fresh and raw fruits and vegetables, get proper rest, good exercise, clean air, fresh water, relax and take it easy, always trusting in our Heavenly Father who wants only the best for us.

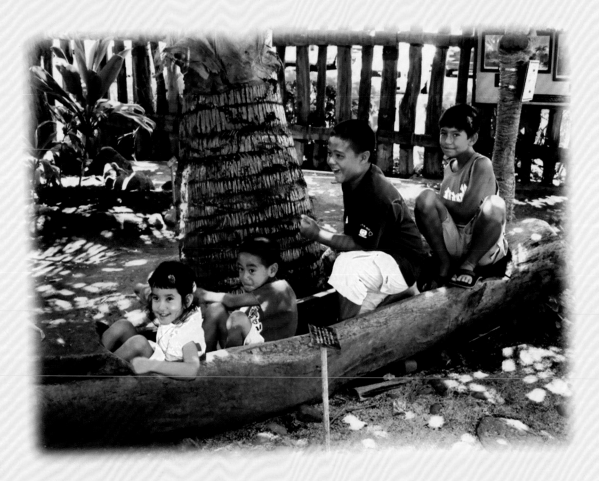

Currently, cows are being injected with a bovine growth hormone (rBGH) that is thought to indirectly increase milk production by stimulating another hormone called Insulin-Like Growth Factor 1, or IGF-1. This hormone is not destroyed by pasteurization. Humans naturally have the exact same IGF-1 hormone in their bodies so, every time people drink milk from an rBGH-injected cow, they increase the amount of active IGF-1 hormones in their system, among other things. Cows injected with rBGH are more likely to develop an infection of the udder known as mastitis, causing pus to accumulate in their milk. The infection must then be treated with antibiotics that also end up in their milk along with the pus and the IGF-1 hormone.

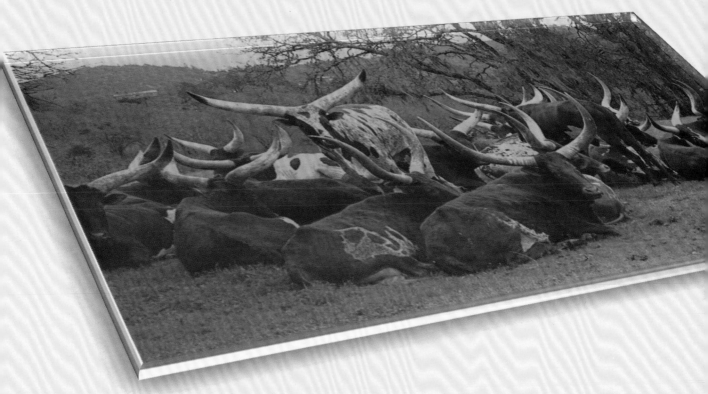

What could an increase of a hormone that stimulates cell production mean to the average person? There in fact, have been many studies that link higher levels of IGF-1 hormones to the increased risk of cancer. Many people continue to use dairy in their diet. I did until I found out what really goes into it.   Throughout this book, we will use the term "milk" which nowadays can come from various sources such as nuts: cashews, almonds, hazelnuts, etc., seeds: sunflower, hemp, etc.,   grains: brown rice, oats, etc., and coconut. Experiment with the different ingredients and combinations. Learn the "mouth feel" and taste each produces. Use those that produce the results you like for the recipe you are working with. In creating your own milks, you can adjust them from thick and rich crèmes for topping desserts, to flavorful milks for cereal. Our recipes are not set in stone. We encourage you to use them as a guide to make your own creations.

"PAA KAI"-Salt from the Sea.

We all know already that our body is 75% water, not all of us know is that this water contained in all of our tissues, cells, blood, etc. is a salty water solution, very similar to the seawater. Another point of interest is that the first 9 months of our lives is spent in a salt water solution.
It does not raise the blood pressure. It is the insufficiency of other minerals that normally hold on to and keep water inside the cells that causes a rise in blood pressure. Given in conjunction with other minerals, salt will actually lower blood pressure to normal levels. Salt can be very effective in stabilizing irregular heartbeats and, contrary to the misconception that it causes high blood pressure (in conjunction with water and the other essential minerals).One or two glasses of water with a little salt will quickly and efficiently quiet the racing and "thumping" heart and, in the long run, will reduce the blood pressure. Salt is a strong antihistamine. It can be used to release asthma. Put it on the tongue after drinking a glass or two of water. It is as effective as an inhaler, without the toxicity. It can also stop persistent dry cough and clear the lungs of mucus plugs and sticky

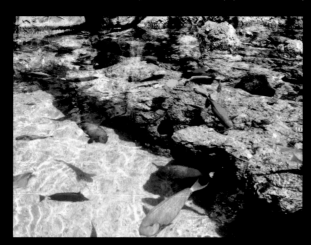

phlegm, particularly in asthma, emphysema and cystic fibrosis sufferers. Salt is vital for extracting excess acidity from inside the cells, particularly the brain cells. Salt is vital for the kidneys to clear excess acidity and pass the acidity to the urine. Without it the body will become more and more acidic, and a strong anti stress element for the body. It is essential in the treatment of emotional and effective disorders. Lithium is a salt substitute that is used in the treatment of depression.

Genuinely healthful sea salt is composed of minerals from the ocean waters which have been transformed by microorganisms, algae and plants into organic nutrients. These, in turn, are bio-available to creatures of the sea and land. Trace elements are found in minute quantities in sea water and therefore in natural unrefined sea salt. They seem to be absent in an Organic Health regime but they all work together to assure and maintain proper function of the body's systems. If any one of them is left out -or even just diminished- a link will be missing, and the whole organism will suffer as a result. Stated another way, if any of our internal oceans are shortchanged of trace nutrients, the body will lack the triggering bio-electrical impulses and the mineral building blocks necessary to function at full efficiency or to renew its systems properly. Salt is vital for the prevention and treatment of the cancer. Cancer cells - When the body is well hydrated and salt expends the volume of blood circulation to reach all parts of the body, the oxygen and active immune cells in the blood reach the cancerous tissue and destroy it. Salt is also important for sleep regulation - it is a natural hypnotic
drink a full glass of water, then put a few grains of salt on your tongue and let it stay there, you will fall into a natural, deep sleep. Salt is a vitally needed element for diabetics. It helps balance the sugar levels in the blood and reduces the need of insulin. Scientific research reveals that there are actually very few salt-related health problems, especially when using unrefined Celtic Sea Salt. A healthy, active lifestyle demands a sufficient reasonable salt intake. The contention that our body can function on no salt at all or on a restricted ration of salt causes more problems than it is intended to solve! Most often, salt-related health problems are caused by diets consisting of high quantities of refined sodium compounds, combined with a sedentary lifestyle.

Sea salt is found in the form of fine or coarse grain, and contains more than a 100 minerals in it. Sea salt and refined salt have the same nutritional value, but they differ in their taste and texture. Table salt is obtained from the rock salt that is mined from mineral deposits. Due to the variations in their refining processes, both salts differ in taste and texture. The end product after refining either of the salts is sodium chloride, which is necessary for the body to function properly. According to experts, recommended intake of sodium should be somewhere between 1,500 and 2,300 milligrams per day, for healthy adults. Hence, some people prefer using sea salt in their food as it has a more subtle flavor. Since the underground salt deposits that produce most table salt are the result of evaporating seawater or salty lakes, you'd think the chemistry would be pretty much the same, and mostly it is. Both rock salt and sea salt contain, besides sodium chloride, such chemicals as calcium, potassium, and magnesium sulfates. However, when a large body of water evaporates, the chemicals in it precipitate out in stages - calcium compounds get deposited first, then sodium, and finally magnesium and potassium. Because of this, a rock salt deposit is often a more homogenous mass of sodium chloride than what you get by drying out seawater commercially. Since rock salt destined for human consumption is typically processed to remove grit and other impurities, by the time it reaches the shaker table salt is nearly pure sodium chloride. Sea salt generally is far from pure - the impurities are its big selling point and frequently an identifying mark, such as the tiny bits of clay that give gray sea salt its color, or the iron-rich red volcanic clay added to Hawaiian sea salt. Although fans tout sea salt's trace elements, the major constituents are the aforesaid calcium, potassium, etc. The importance of minerals in the diet can't be dismissed; after all, the iodine commonly added to table salt helps prevent thyroid conditions. But there's little (actually, from what I can tell, no) research demonstrating that consuming sea salt is helpful in ways that consuming the ordinary kind isn't. Conceivably a benefit will someday be shown; for example, a few studies claim mineral-rich Dead Sea water - when bathed in, not drunk - is useful in treating psoriasis. Sea salt is beneficial to the skin. Skin absorbs sea salts, vitamins and any other substances it comes into contact with. It is universally accepted that sea salts can have a wonderful effect on circulation and metabolism. Sea salts contain many minerals beneficial to the body. Magnesium is important for combating stress and fluid retention, slowing skin aging and calming the nervous system. Calcium is effective at preventing water retention, increasing circulation and strengthening bones and nails. Potassium energizes the body, helps to balance skin moisture and is a crucial mineral to replenish after intense exercise. Bromides act to ease muscle stiffness and relax muscles. Sodium is important for lymphatic fluid balance (this is important for the immune system).So we can see that bathing in high quality sea salts could replenish the minerals vital to our skin metabolism. Medical research also shows that the high blood pressure problem lies not in salt intake but in an overactive hormone system. Sea Salt can actually help you lower your blood pressure. The Creator created our bodies to need salt. Whenever a recipe calls for salt, we prefer using sea salt. Celtic Sea Salt is our favorite brand which can be found in natural foods markets or in your grocers' natural foods aisle. . A word to the wise, let's do some homework and find out what kinds of salt will best work for our bodies and don't just take my word for it. Please research it on your own as well.

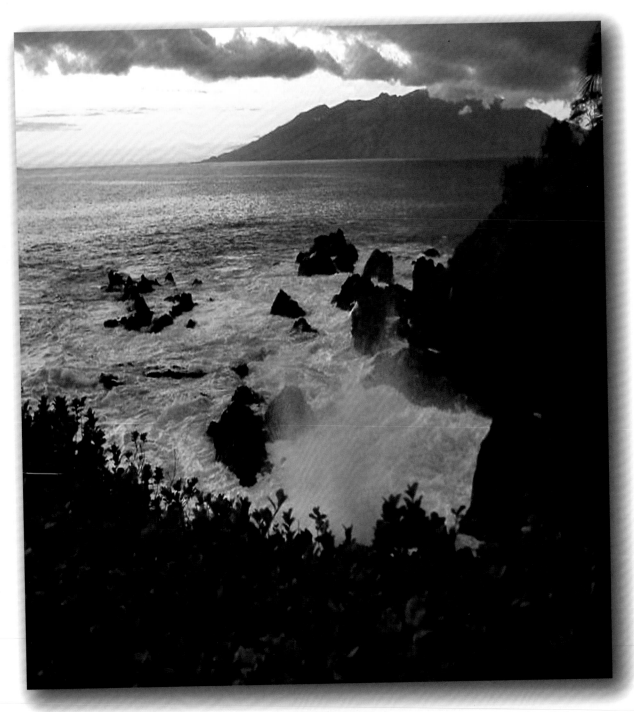

Although it may seem like you're seeing another island, it is really the west side of the same island, as Maui can be compared to a figure-8 shape. There, you can hike a 5.5 mile trail from one side to the other. This place is called NA PALI- the Cliffs. Fabulous for watching the Humpback whales, they frequent this bay with their calves because of its calm waters.

Tools

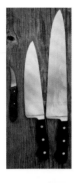

You will want to get good knives because they will make your life much easier in the kitchen. They need to be kept sharp and clean which will help you get the work done with less effort. Look for knives that have the blade going all the way through the handle. Knives made this way are best for giving strength and balance. The little one on the far left of the photo is a tourne knife, great for peeling and for small jobs. The larger ones are German-made knives in 10" and 12" lengths.

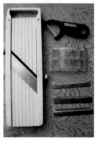

The tool pictured here is a mandolin that we like to use. With three interchangeable blades, it is limitless in use and a must-have tool in food production. Use a mandolin for the recipes that call for finely sliced or julienned vegetables. You can find this particular brand called Benriner inexpensively in many Asian markets. Don't forget your peeler. We like the style of the one in the top right corner of this photo. But any quality one will do.

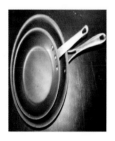

These Teflon-coated non-stick pans are my preference. Although some may be concerned about the Teflon coating, I believe it only becomes harmful once the coating begins to flake off, making it ingestible. Please don't use metal tongs, spatulas or anything else that could cause that to happen. These pans are great for cutting the amount oil you use in food production.

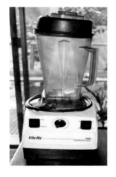

A high speed blender is very nice to have. Ones like the Vitamix shown here may be pricey, but well worth the ticket. Not only does it do the obvious, but it can make flour from whole grains and is great for emulsifying products. The speed alone allows you to omit some binders.

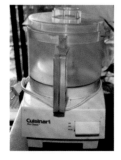

Food processors: every kitchen needs one. They are the greatest time saver and worth the small investment if you do a lot of cooking. With so many on the market to choose from, I would suggest you do your homework and get a good one that will last.

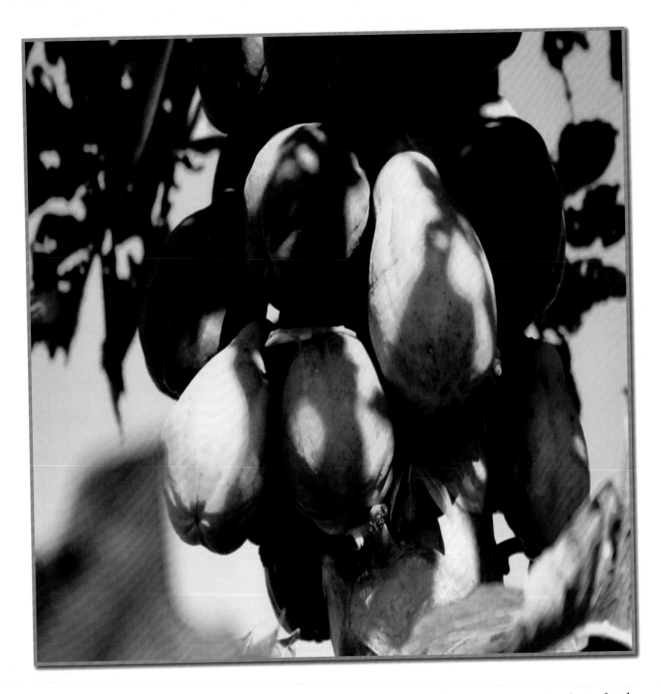

Papaya is one of many exotic plants we find in the islands with diverse uses ranging from food consumption to beauty care and even rope making. The enzymes of the papaya are beneficial for applying to Portuguese man-o-war and jellyfish stings, as they tend to break down the proteins from the animal. You can see in the photo above humans are not the only one that likes the fruit. This little guy is happy to have the cool shade of the papaya tree.

Appetizers

Boiled Peanuts

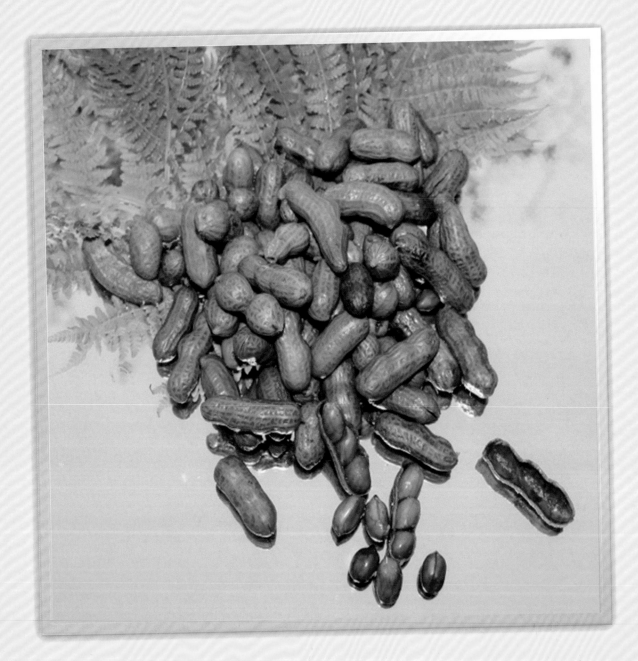

Peanuts, which are usually consumed in ways similar to tree nuts, are actually in the legume family and grow underground. They contain more fat and fewer carbohydrates than of the other legumes.

Boiled Peanuts

2 lb dry peanuts

1 gallon water

½ cup sea salt

Sort and rinse peanuts and place in a stock pot with the water and salt. Bring to a boil, and then reduce heat to medium, keeping it at a low boil. The cooking time may take up to eight hours. Check occasionally after the first hour of cooking.

Another cooking method that I like to use is after bringing the water to a boil, reduce the heat to low and continue to cook for two hours. After two hours, turn off the heat and let it sit out for another 6-8 hours (or overnight). The following day, bring it to a boil once again. Reduce the heat to a low boil and check after 1 hour and every hour after that until peanuts are soft, but not mushy. About 4 hours.

Once the peanuts are cooked, drain, cool down and store in a container in the refrigerator. This is a favorite snack among many in Hawaii.

For an Asian-flavored version, add three or four **star anise** pods to the water.

Star Anise Broiled Japanese Eggplant

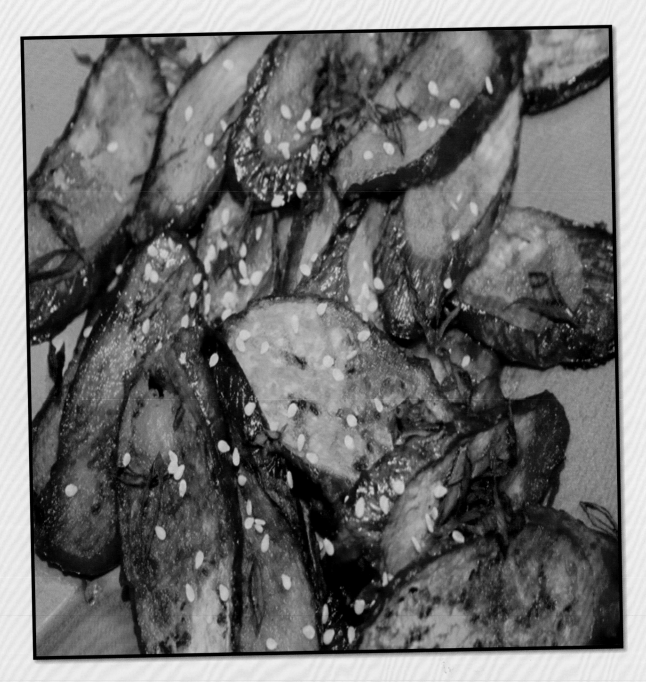

Eggplant skin is called Nasunin. It is a potent antioxidant and free radical scavenger that has been shown to protect cell membranes from damage. Try to find fresh eggplant; best place is from your yard. The skins shouldn't be too bitter or tough, peel them if they are.

Star Anise Broiled Japanese Eggplant

3 Japanese eggplants

2 Tbsp. each olive oil and sesame oil mix together

2 Tbsp finely sliced basil or 1 tsp. dried basil

3 Tbsp nutritional yeast

2 Tbsp garlic chopped fine

1/8 to ¼ tsp. star anise powder

3 Tbsp almond butter

Cut off stem and discard. Slice eggplant on bias (diagonal) ¼ inch thick, sprinkle with salt and let sit in a colander for one hour. Rinse thoroughly with water. Drain the excess liquid and pat dry with paper towels. Set aside.

Combine the oils, basil, nutritional yeast, garlic, star anise powder and almond butter in a bowl, whisk to incorporate the ingredients. Dip the eggplant slices into the mixture, coating each side. Lay slices on a sheet pan. Place the eggplant in the oven and broil on high. Check after 5-8 minutes. Once browned, remove from oven and use a spatula to turn over. Set it back in the oven and brown the other side, 5-8 minutes.

Arrange on serving platter and garnish with chopped green onions and sesame seeds. Serve immediately or keep in a warm oven until ready to serve.

Glazed Onion Stuffed with Curried Vegetable

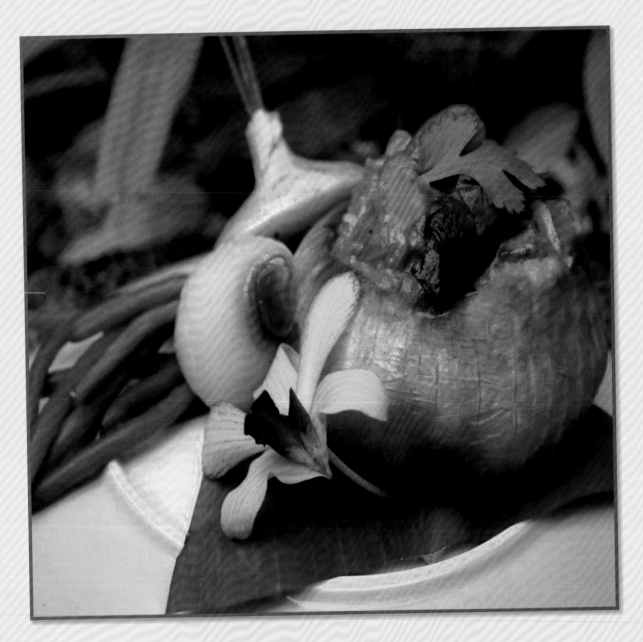

The higher the intake of onion, the lower the level of glucose found during oral or intravenous glucose tolerance tests. In addition, onions are a very good source of chromium, the mineral component in glucose tolerance factor, a molecule that helps cells respond appropriately to insulin. Raw onions sliced and placed on bleeding wounds help to stop the bleeding.

Glazed Onion Stuffed with Curried Vegetable

4 large white onions

1 Tbsp olive oil

¼ cup garlic chopped

8 shiitake mushrooms, remove stems and dice

1 red bell pepper diced

1 stalk celery diced

2 onions diced

1 tsp sea salt or to taste

3 Tbsp curry mix p.142

¼ cup mango chutney

6 oz coconut milk

8 oz tomato juice or vegetable juice

¼ cup fresh cilantro chopped

To prepare the glazed onion: trim the top and the bottom, do not remove the skin. Rub the skins with olive oil and place on a sheet pan. Brown in the oven at 450 degrees, 15-20 minutes. Remove from the oven. Use a spoon to scoop out the center portion of the onion, creating a cavity just large enough to be filled with the vegetable mixture and yet not too thin that it will collapse. You can use the center for garnish or dice it up and add to the vegetable filling. Set aside the onions until ready to fill.

In a large skillet over medium heat, add the oil and garlic. Sauté for one minute. Add in the mushrooms, celery, diced onions, garlic and salt. Sprinkle in curry spice, and stir the spices with the vegetables until fragrant, one minute. Reduce the heat to low. In a bowl, mix the mango chutney, coconut milk and tomato or vegetable juice. Add this to the skillet and stir to combine. Continue to simmer on low for 5-8 minutes.

To the skillet, add the cilantro in the last few minutes of cooking. Remove from heat and allow to cool slightly. Spoon the filling into the onion cavities and place on a baking dish. Keep warm in oven or serve immediately.

Summer Vegetable Hashbrown

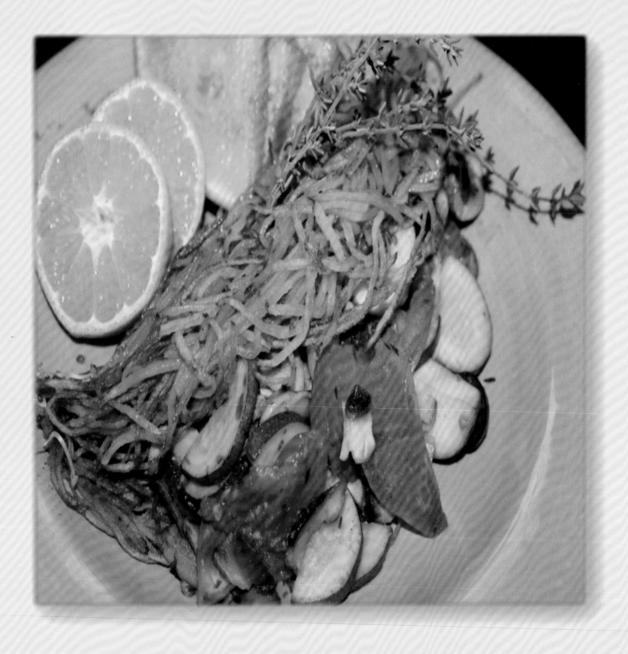

White potatoes can offer many health benefits. They contain nutrition and small quantities of atropine. It is essentially used to combat gastrointestinal pain and cramping. The old folk medicines used the potato to apply externally for muscle pain and other skin problems. If the potato is applied to your joint and muscles, it should be warm. It also improves circulation if applied externally.

Summer Vegetable Hashbrown

2 large russet potato

1 tsp tumeric

1/8 tsp paprika

1 tsp garlic powder

1 tsp sea salt or to taste

olive oil

1 medium zuccini – sliced

½ white onion–sliced

8 button mushrooms–sliced

½ tomato sliced

fresh herbs thyme,or basil

1 Tbsp chopped garlic

Peel and grate the potato the night before and soak in water, place in refrigerator. When ready for use, drain the liquid out. Mix in the tumeric, paprika, garlic powder and salt. Let sit for a few minutes till it gets to room temperature. In a non-stick skillet, heat a teaspoon of oil. Take half a handful of the potato mixture and spread over the surface of pan thinly. Brown on both sides. After all the potatoes have been cooked, set aside.

In the same pan, add a teaspoon oil and garlic, stirring until browned. Toss in the remaining vegetables. Saute until tender– at this point you may add in any other type of your favorite seasoning or flavor combination. Cook till tender, remove from heat.

Place each potato hashbrown on a serving dish and fill with the vegetables. Fold over and serve.

Oven Roasted Roma Tomato

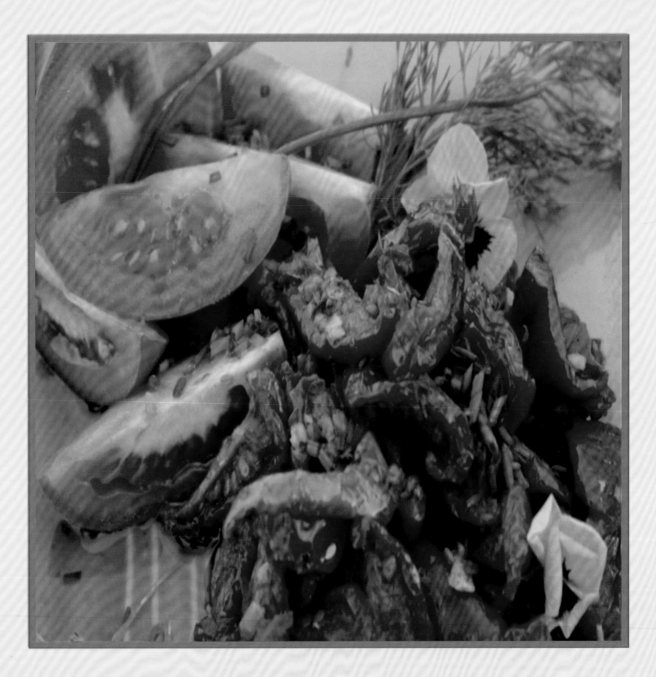

Organic ketchup delivers three times as much of the cancer-fighting carotenoid, lycopene, as non-organic brands. Lycopene has been shown to help protect not only against prostate, but breast, pancreatic and intestinal cancers, especially when consumed with fat-rich foods, such as avocado, olive oil or nuts.

Oven Roasted Roma Tomato

24 ripe Roma or plum tomatoes

8 cloves garlic chopped

¼ cup equal parts of fresh dill, parsley, basil and chives

½ cup olive oil

sea salt to taste

Quarter tomatoes and place them in a large mixing bowl. Set aside.

In a blender, combine garlic, herbs and olive oil, processing until smooth. Pour the oil mixture into the bowl with the tomatoes. Stir to coat them well.

Lay tomatoes in a single layer on a sheet pan and sprinkle with sea salt.

Place the tomatoes in the oven at lowest possible temperature. It may take up to ten hours of cooking time, check and rotate the sheet pans occasionally. Tomatoes are done when they have shrunk considerably.

Store with the oil in a glass jar in the refrigerator for up to 2 weeks or place in thick plastic bags and freeze. Having these tomatoes are great for adding to soups, sauces, salads, casseroles, etc.

Togorashi Pepper Mung Bean Sprouts

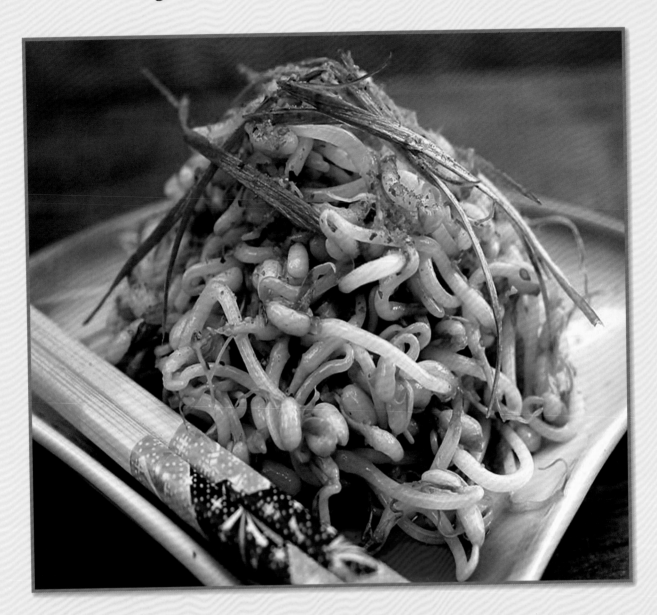

Used extensively in Asian cuisine, bean sprouts are not often considered by the public as a nutritional element. However, bean sprouts, or rather Mung Bean sprouts, as they are properly called, contain pure forms of vitamins A, B, C, and E, in addition to an assortment of minerals including Calcium, Iron, and Potassium.

Togorashi Pepper Mung Bean Sprouts

2 cups mung bean sprouts rinsed

1 Tbsp garlic sliced

2 Tbsp sesame oil

2 Tbsp soy sauce

Togarashi Pepper to taste

4 green onions sliced thin on the bias

In a non stick skillet over medium-low heat, add the sesame oil and garlic. Slowly brown the garlic. Once the garlic is soft and golden brown, increase the heat to medium-high. Drop in bean sprouts, cooking until wilted, about two minutes. Do not overcook, sprouts should be wilted and yet crisp.

Drizzle the soy sauce and remove to a serving plate. To garnish, sprinkle with Japanese Togarashi pepper and green onions.

Involtini con i Legumi

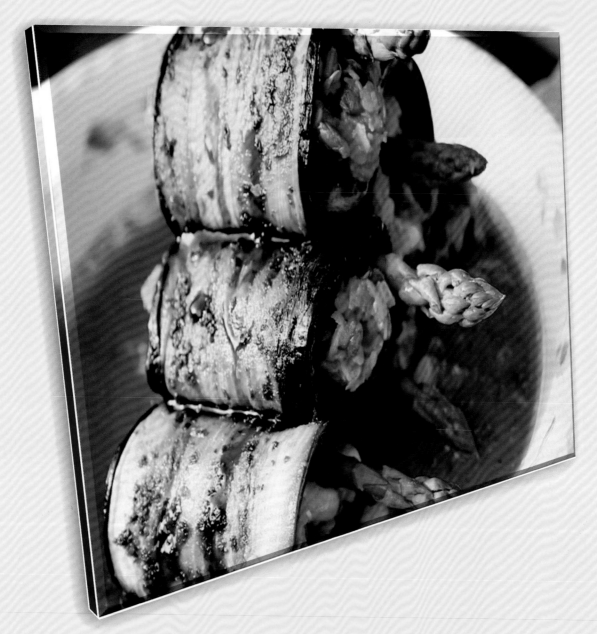

Involtini, small Italian rolls, here are combined with legumes. Legumes contain relatively low quantities of the essential amino acid methionine. That is why most vegetarian cultures - in order to get a balanced diet, and almost in an involuntary manner - combine their diet of legumes with grains. Grains, on the other hand, contain relatively low quantities of the essential amino acid lysine, which legumes contain. Serve this main dish with a healthy portion of whole grains such as quinoa or brown rice.

Involtini con i Legumi

2 large eggplants

2/3 cup dry navy beans, soaked overnight

2/3 cup dry green lentils

2/3 cup dry red lentils

Cut off stem and end of the eggplant and slice lengthwise ¼". Sprinkle with salt and allow it to sit in a colander for one hour.

Rinse beans separately in a colander and place each in a separate pot. Cover with water and bring to a boil. Reduce heat to medium and simmer until cooked. Navy beans take the longest to cook, while the red lentils take the least amount of time to cook. Once cooked, drain and place all the legumes in one bowl. Set aside.

3 Tbsp annatto-infused oil	2 Tbsp molasses
½ onion diced fine	1 - 14 oz can stewed tomato
¼ green bell pepper diced fine	sea salt to taste
½ celery stalk diced fine	1 Tbsp garlic minced
12 asparagus spears blanched and cooled	

In a sauce pan over medium-high heat, add the infused oil, onions, pepper, celery, and garlic. Sauté until tender and brown. Add the molasses and tomatoes. Simmer for ten minutes, adding salt to taste. Remove from heat and carefully blend until smooth.

Slowly add some of the sauce to the legumes, adding just enough to bind the ingredients together. Keep the remaining sauce on the side for serving.

Rinse the eggplant with water and pat dry with paper towels. Lay each slice on a flat surface. Place 2 Tbsp of the mixture at the top edge of the eggplant and roll towards the other edge. Insert an asparagus spear in the middle and continue to roll to the other edge. Lay involtini on a baking sheet or dish and broil until the eggplant is browned. Reduce temperature to 350 degrees and allow the rolls to continue to warm, about 10 minutes. Arrange on a plate and serve with the extra sauce.

Makes approximately 10-14 rolls.

Saffron Stuffed Potato Dumplings

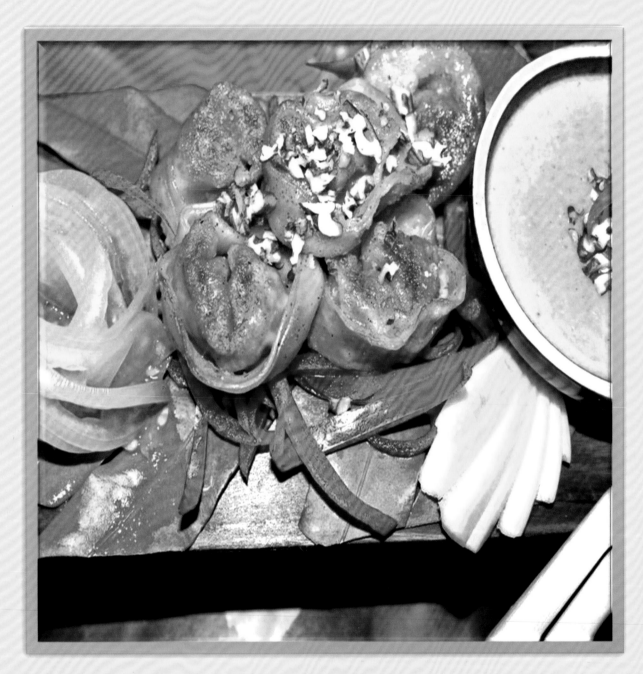

Saffron contains more than 150 volatile and aroma-yielding compounds. It also has many nonvolatile active components many of which are carotenoids, including zeaxanthin, lycopene and various A- and β-carotenes. However, saffron's golden yellow-orange colour is primarily the result of A-crocin. Saffron is the world's most expensive spice by weight.

Saffron Stuffed Potato Dumplings

3 large russet potatoes

4 cloves garlic fine chop

1 med onion fine dice

6-8 strands of saffron

sea salt to taste

1 Tbsp olive oil

2 Tbsp cilantro chopped fine

wonton wrappers

2 Tbsp chopped pecans

1 Tbsp sesame oil

1 Tbsp chopped garlic

2 Tbsp curry mix pg 142

¼ cup coconut milk

1 Tbsp finely chopped green onion

Coconut milk for sauce—1/4 cup per serving 8 pieces per serving.

Soak stands of saffron in ¼ cup coconut milk the night before and refrigerate.

In a saucepan, bring water and potatoes to a boil. Boil for 5 minutes then reduce heat to a low boil and cook for about 20 minutes or until knife pierces the flesh easily. Drain and cool until easily handled. Peel the skin and use a ricer for the potatoes or a masher to achieve a smooth consistency. Set aside in a large bowl.

In a skillet over medium-high heat, add the oil. To the oil, add the onions and garlic, cooking until translucent. Remove from heat and add to the bowl with potatoes. Pour the saffron/coconut milk mixture into the bowl. Using the masher once again, incorporate all the ingredients.

Place about a teaspoon of the saffron potato filling on the center of a wonton wrapper. Run water along the edges with your fingers to seal and fold in half into a triangle while squeezing out any air. Bend back middle corner and bring the outer corners together in the front, using a dab of water to hold them together. Set on a tray sprinkled with cornstarch. Proceed with remaining wrappers and filling.

To cook the dumplings heat oil in a sauté pan over medium-high heat. Carefully add the dumplings and brown each side. Once browned, add the curry seasoning and pecans, toasting until fragrant, 30 seconds. Pour in the coconut milk and add in the cilantro. Stir to combine. Reduce the liquid until thickened, adding salt to taste. Garnish with green onions and serve immediately.

Alternately, the sauce may be made separately from the dumplings and then poured over the cooked dumplings or set aside as a dipping sauce.

This recipe makes approximately 40-50 pieces which can be frozen for later use.

Luau-Style Sweet Potato

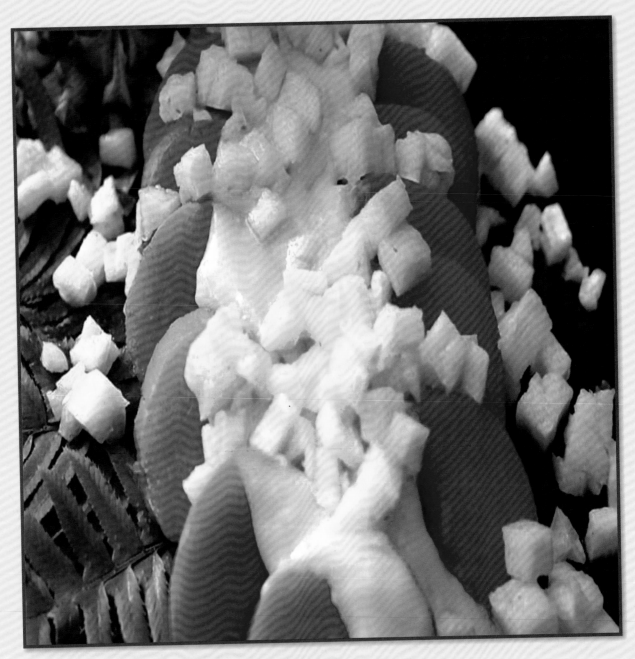

Sweet potato, along with taro, was a major staple of the early Hawaiians. Sweet potatoes are rich in complex carbohydrates, dietary fiber, beta carotene (a vitamin A equivalent nutrient), vitamin C. Pink and yellow varieties are high in carotene, the precursor of vitamin A. Despite the name "sweet", it may be a beneficial food for diabetics, as preliminary studies on animals have revealed that it helps to stabilize blood sugar levels and to lower insulin resistance.

Luau-Style Sweet Potato

2 large yams and/or sweet potato

4 oz coconut milk

2 Tbsp cornstarch mixed with 2 Tbsp water

2 Tbsp agave or organic cane sugar

½ fresh pineapple diced small

Heat oven to 350 degrees. Rinse the yams and/or sweet potaoes and place them on a baking sheet into the oven. Bake for 30 –35 minutes. Check for doneness by inserting a sharp knife in the center. When it is easily pierced, they are done. Remove from the oven and cool until you are able to handle them comfortably. Remove the skins and slice ½" thick. Arrange slices on a dish.

In a sauce pan over medium heat, add the coconut milk and sweetener. While stirring with a whisk, bring to a boil and add the cornstarch mixture to thicken. Once thickened, pour over the yams.   Garnish with the diced fresh pineapple.

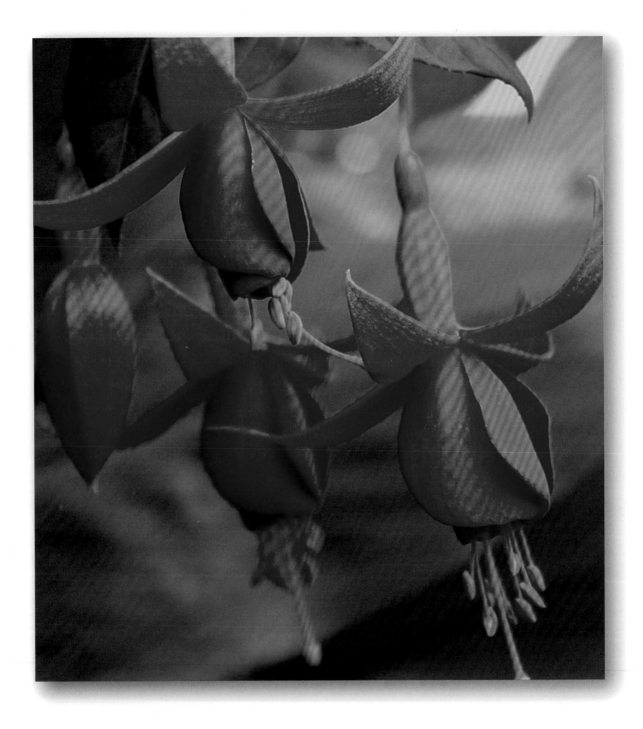

Fuchsia is included in a number of popular garden plants. They come in many different colors and varieties. They're also characterized by flowers with usually four sepals and petals; in some genera, the sepals are as brightly colored as the petals, giving the impression of a flower with eight petals.

Soups

Creamy Asparagus Soup

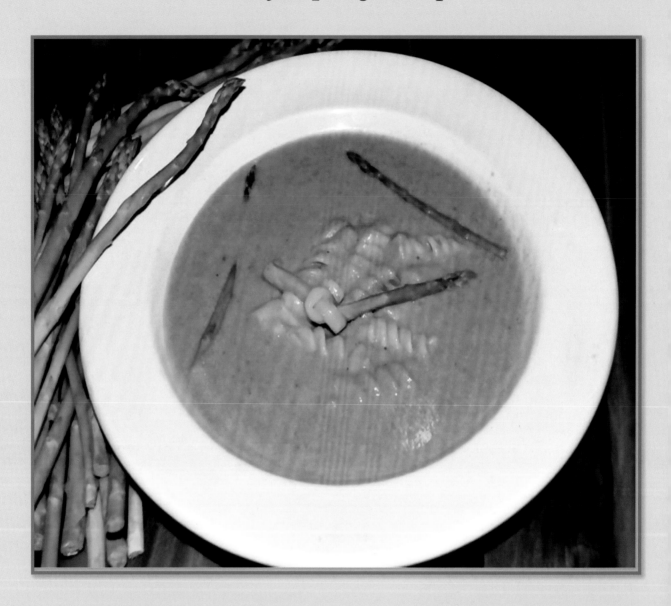

A cup of asparagus supplies approximately 263 mcg of folate, a B-vitamin essential for proper cellular division because it is necessary in DNA synthesis. Without folate, the fetus' nervous system cells do not divide properly. Inadequate folate during pregnancy has been linked to several birth defects, including neural tube defects like spina bifida.

Creamy Asparagus Soup

2 large potatoes, baked

1 Tbsp olive oil

1 medium onion, small dice

1 carrot, small dice

2 ribs celery, small dice

1 Tbsp chopped garlic

2 lbs. asparagus

3 cups water

½ cup milk

½ cup cashews

1 cup whole grain pasta, cooked

sea salt to taste

Set aside several spears of asparagus for garnishing. Blanch or broil the asparagus spears and set aside. Cut the remaining asparagus into ½ '' pieces.

Remove skins from the cooled baked potato. Dice and set aside.

In saucepan on medium–high heat, add oil and brown the onion, carrot, celery, garlic and the cut asparagus. Sauté until browned and tender.   Add the water, milk, potatoes and cashews. Reduce heat and simmer for 10 minutes.

Carefully ladle the soup into blender cup. Cover with the lid and process until smooth. Use caution when blending to prevent accidents. Pour the soup back into the saucepan and keep heat at low. Stir in the pasta. When ready to serve, ladle into serving bowls and garnish with the asparagus spears. Makes about 1 quart.

Roasted Garlic

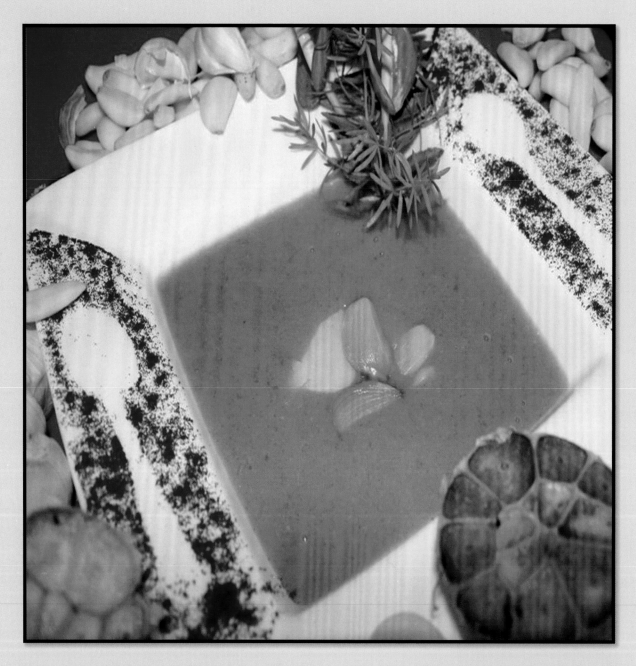

Garlic has long been considered an herbal "wonder drug", with a reputation in folklore for preventing everything from the common cold and flu to the Plague! In general, a stronger tasting clove of garlic has more sulphur content and hence more medicinal value. Modern science has shown that garlic is a powerful natural antibiotic, albeit broad-spectrum rather than targeted.

Roasted Garlic

2 whole bulbs of roasted garlic

1 Tbsp olive oil

1 Tbsp garlic rough cut

1 medium onion small dice

1 rib of celery rough cut

½ carrot peeled and rough cut

1 Tbsp paprika

2 ½ cups water

1/3 cup cashews

2 med potatoes

1 cup coconut milk

½ tsp sea salt

Cut the root end off whole garlic bulb; place on a sheet pan in oven for 20 minutes at 300 degrees or till soft. Squeeze out garlic cloves from the cut end when cooled and set aside.

Place oil in a saucepan on medium–high heat. Add the onion, garlic, celery and carrots. Brown the vegetables.

Add paprika cook for another minute, stirring to prevent scorching. Add water and potatoes, simmer until potatoes softened.

In a blender, carefully add the roasted garlic and sautéed vegetables with the cashews and coconut milk. Process until smooth.   Replace to the same saucepan and turn heat to low. Add salt to taste and continue to simmer for 30 minutes more on low heat. Makes approximately 1 quart.

Hawaiian Hot and Sour

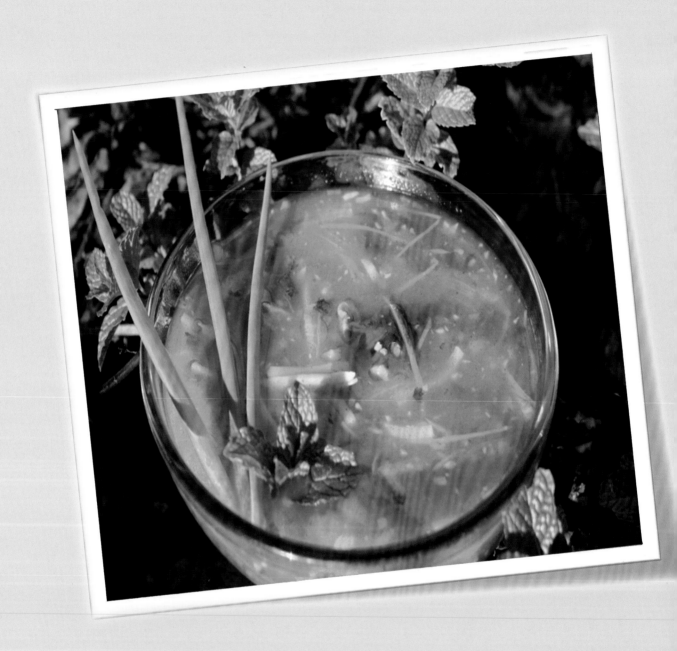

Red chilies are very high in potassium and high in magnesium and iron. Capsaicin is a safe and effective analgesic agent in the management of arthritis pain, herpes zoster-related pain, diabetic neuropathy, post mastectomy pain, and headaches. Red chilies contain high amounts of vitamin C and carotene.

Hawaiian Hot and Sour

2 Tbsp sesame oil

3 Tbsp garlic chopped fine

3 Tbsp fine ginger chopped fine

3 ribs of celery julienne

1 ½ cup onion

2 whole carrots julienne

3 tsp sea salt

1 cup dries shiitake mushroom in 2 cups water

½ tsp red chili flakes

½ cup cilantro rough cut

8 oz bamboo shoots strips

¾ cup sushi vinegar or lime juice

1 ½ quarts pineapple juice

8 oz straw mushroom in water

2 tsp paprika

¼ cup cornstarch to ¼ cup water

In a saucepan on low heat, infuse the garlic and ginger in oil for 3 three minutes.

Increase the heat to high and add onion, carrots, and celery. Cook until translucent, 3–5 minutes.

Stir in paprika. Add the remaining ingredients and bring to rapid boil.

Reduce heat to low and simmer for 20 minutes. Adjust with salt and thicken with cornstarch/water mixture.

Serve piping hot. Makes 2 quarts.

Vegetable and Leek

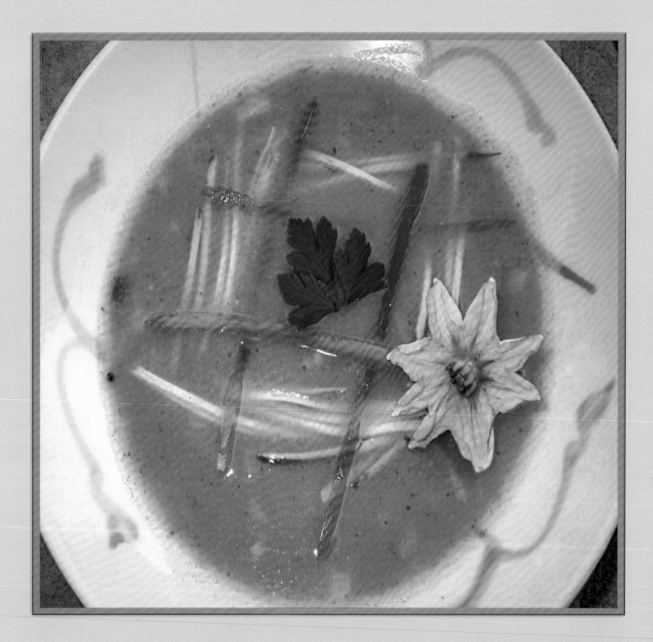

Easier to digest than standard onions, leeks have laxative, antiseptic, diuretic, and anti-arthritic properties. They not only slow the absorption of sugars from the intestinal tract, but help ensure that they are properly metabolized in the body.

Vegetable and Leek

1 Tbsp olive oil

1 large onion diced

2 ribs of celery diced

½ bulb garlic peeled

1 large leek diced

1 head of broccoli

4 cups water

2 large russets peeled and small diced

1 Tbsp fresh rosemary

2 Tbsp fresh parsley

sea salt to taste

In a large stock pot, heat the oil over high. Add the garlic cloves, onions, celery, bell pepper, leek, and broccoli. Sauté until they become tender and brown in color.

Pour in water and add the potatoes.

Bring to rapid boil then simmer for 15 minutes. At this point add the herbs.

Remove from heat and carefully blend until smooth. Pour back into the pot and adjust with salt if needed. Makes 1 quart.

Black Bean Soup w/Avocado Crème

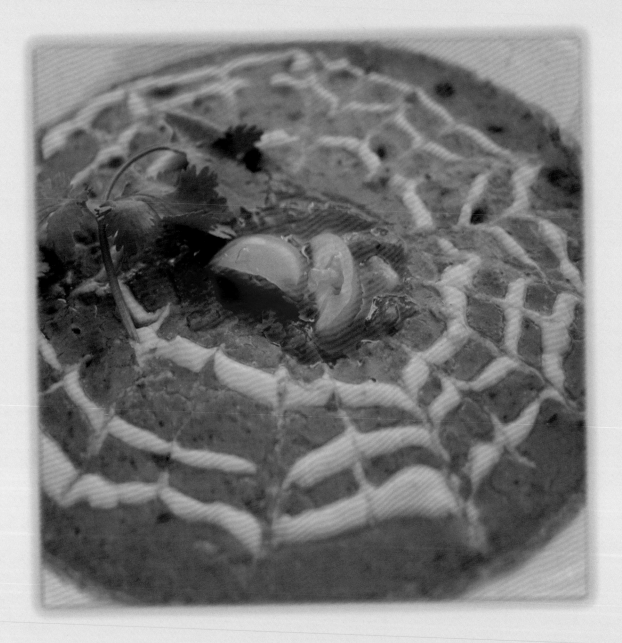

Black beans are as rich in antioxidant compounds called anthocyanins as grapes and cranberries, fruits long considered antioxidant superstars. In addition to its beneficial effects on the digestive system and the heart, black beans' soluble fiber helps stabilize blood sugar levels. If you have insulin resistance, hypoglycemia or diabetes, black beans can really help you balance blood sugar levels while providing steady, slow-burning energy.

Black Bean Soup w/Avocado Crème

1 Tbsp olive oil	1 tsp paprika
½ onion diced medium	½ tsp cumin
½ green bell pepper diced medium	½ tsp curry powder
1 Tbsp chopped garlic	½ tsp fresh or ground oregano
12 oz. black beans cooked and drained	¼ cup sliced green onion
1 tomato diced	½ cup chopped cilantro
water	sea salt to taste

Heat oil in a saucepan over medium-high heat. Add the onion, bell pepper, and garlic. Sauté until tender.

Sprinkle in the paprika, cumin, curry powder and oregano and cook in the spices for another few minutes.

Stir in the cooked and drained black beans, green onion, and tomato. Simmering over medium-low heat.

Pour just enough water to cover the beans by one inch and bring to a rapid boil. Simmer for 20 minutes. Add the cilantro in just before blending.

Ladle into a blender and process until smooth. Pour into serving dishes and top with Avocado Crème sauce. Serve immediately.

Avocado Crème.

1 medium avocado, remove pit	¼ cup water
1 Tbsp lemon juice	¼ tsp sea salt
¼ cup raw almonds	1 ½ tsp nutritional yeast
2 Tbsp cilantro	

Place almonds, lemon juice and water in the blender and process until smooth. Add the remaining ingredients and continue blending until smooth and creamy.

Kale and Shiitake

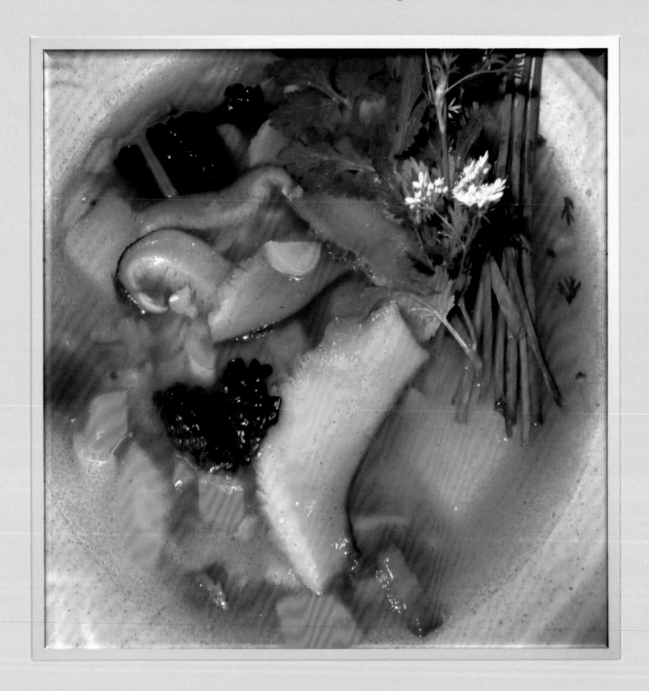

Kale is very high in beta carotene, vitamin k, and vitamin c beta carotene and reasonably rich in calcium. Because of its high vitamin K content, patients taking anti-coagulants are encouraged to avoid this food since it increases the vitamin K concentration in the blood, which is what the drugs are often attempting to lower.

Kale and Shiitake

½ cup dried shiitake mushrooms

1 Tbsp olive oil

1 med onion diced small

1 whole red bell pepper diced small

1 large carrot, med dice

2 gloves garlic, sliced thin

1 Tbsp paprika

1 quart water

2 Tbsp soy sauce

½ cup cooked rice

5 leaves of dinosaur kale, chopped

chipotle paste to taste

sea salt to taste

Soak dried shiitake mushrooms in 1 quart warm water. Set aside.

Heat a stock pot over medium-high heat and add the oil. Place onions, bell pepper, carrots, garlic and paprika, sauté till translucent.

Strain the shiitake mushrooms, reserving the liquid. Pour this liquid into the stock pot. Cut the mushrooms into bite-sized pieces and add to soup. Simmer for 15 minutes.

Add the cooked rice, kale and soy sauce.   Add chipotle paste a little at a time until you achieve the desired spiciness. Makes about 1 quart.

Roasted Beet

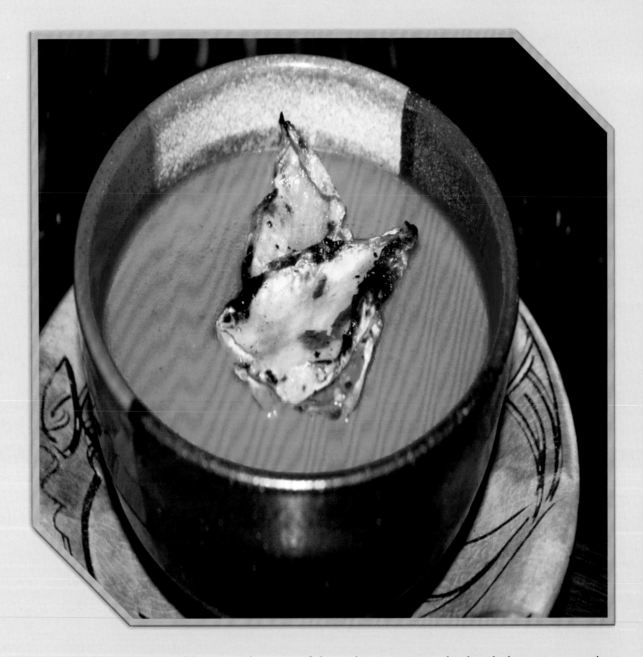

These colorful root vegetables contain powerful nutrient compounds that help protect against heart disease, birth defects and certain cancers, especially colon cancer. Beets are an excellent source of the B vitamin, folate, and a very good source of manganese and potassium. Beets are a good source of dietary fiber, vitamin C, magnesium, iron, copper and phosphorus.

Roasted Beet

½ pound red beets (about 3 medium)

1 ½ tsp olive oil

1 leek (white and pale green parts only) chopped

1 small onion, thinly sliced

1 fresh parsley sprig

1 fresh thyme sprig

¼ cup coconut milk

1/8 tsp ground ginger

1/8 tsp ground allspice

1 small bay leaf

2 cups water

1 rib of celery chopped

1 small bay leaf

sea salt to taste

Wrap beets in foil and roast in an oven at 350 degrees until tender, about 1 hour.   Cool.   Peel and cut beets into ½ inch pieces.   Set aside.

Heat oil in a saucepan over medium–high heat.   Place leek, onion, and celery and cook until beginning to brown, stirring frequently.   Stir in ginger, allspice, white pepper, and ½ inch beet pieces.

Pour in the water and add the bay leaf, thyme, and parsley.   Bring to boil for 5 minutes.   Reduce heat to low, cover, and simmer until vegetables are very tender, about 25 minutes.

Remove bay leaf, thyme sprig, and parsley sprig, puree soup in blender and add coconut milk while blending.

Adjust with salt. Photo is shown garnished with marinated and broiled endive leaves.

Wild Mushroom with Yam Noodle

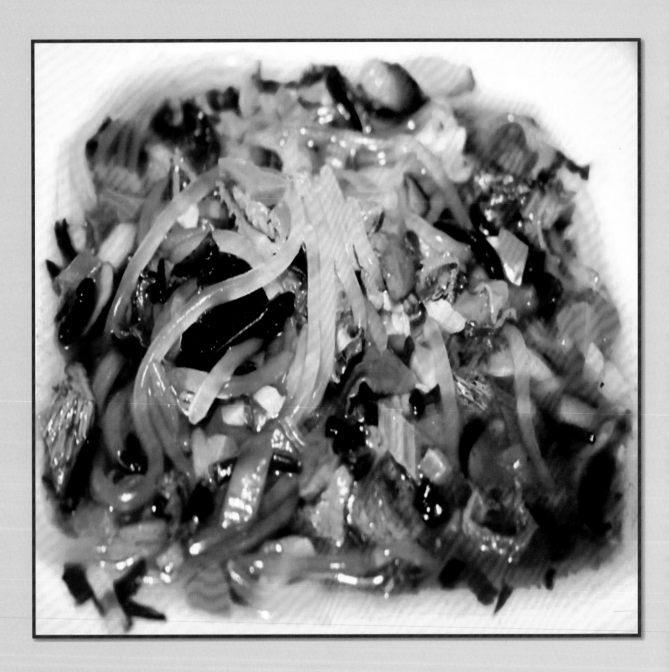

Shirataki is a translucent noodle made from the powdered root of the Asian konjac yam. They consist mostly of a no-calorie, highly soluble fiber called glucomannan. Glucomannan helps lower bad LDL cholesterol, triglycerides, fasting blood sugar, and even body weight. What's more, scientists in Thailand found that just 1 gram has the power to significantly slow the absorption of sugar into your bloodstream after eating a carb-loaded meal.

Wild Mushroom with Yam Noodle

2 Tbsp sesame oil

2 Tbsp chopped garlic

½ onion small dice

1 small carrot small dice

3 celery ribs small dice

¼ green bell pepper small dice

20 strands dry Yam noodle, cut 2–3" lengths

¼ cup cornstarch mixed with ¼ cup water

6 fresh button mushrooms sliced

½ cup dried black chinese mushroom

1 cup dried shiitake mushroom

1 cup dried chanterelle mushrooms

2 Tbsp cilantro chopped fine

sea salt to taste

½ tsp smoked paprika

1 quart warm water

Soak dried mushrooms separately in 1 cup of warm water set aside until it softens.

Heat a stock pot to medium–high heat and add oil. Brown garlic, onion, carrots, celery, bell pepper, and button mushrooms. Stir occasionally to avoid scorching.

Strain liquid from the Shiitake and Chanterelle into stock pot. Chop rather small and add to pot. Strain liquid from black mushrooms and discard. Again, chop small and add to pot. At this point add the remaining water along with the cilantro and smoked paprika. Bring to a rapid boil and simmer for 20 minutes. Add the yam noodles. Once noodles are cooked, thicken with cornstarch/water mixture and adjust with salt.

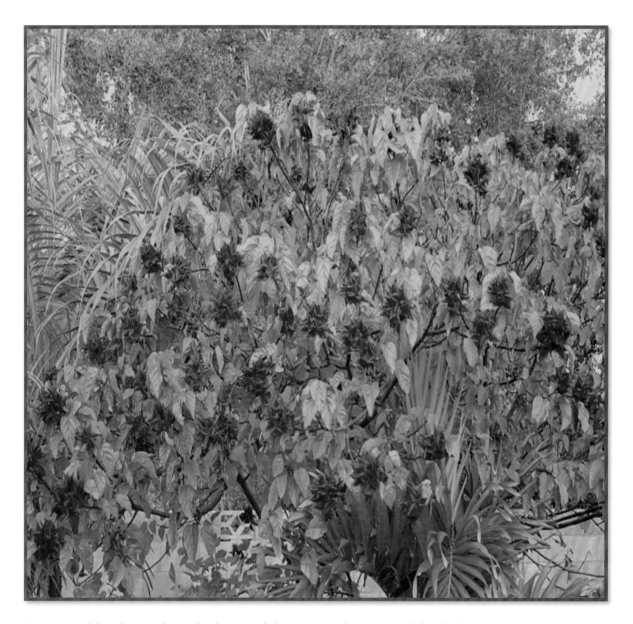

It's a true blessing to have had one of these trees in our yard back in Maui. This is the tree where Achiote or the Annato comes from. There are hard bright red seeds in a spiky outer shell, it doesn't take much to shell them once they're dried. One tree has such high yield that sharing is a moral imperative.

Raw Foods

Butternut Fettuccini

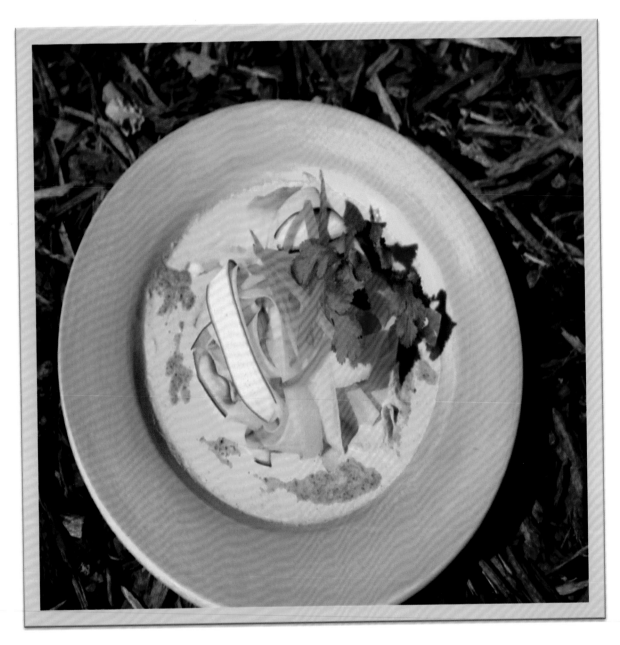

Butternuts are used in soup and can be cooked on a barbecue wrapped in foil with spices such as nutmeg and cinnamon; it is a good source of fiber vitamin C, manganese, magnesium and potassium. It is also an excellent source of vitamin A.

Butternut Fettuccini

1 butternut squash peeled and cut into ½" wide sections

½ zucchini

red bell pepper julienne

Use a mandolin adjusted to the thinnest possible setting with only the straight blade. Shave the butternut squash and the zucchini along its length to form wide strands. These will be the "pasta." Set aside while preparing the sauces.

Sauce Base

½ cup almonds soaked

½ cup sunflower seeds soaked overnight

2 ½–3 cups water

Strain almonds and sunflower seeds, discarding the liquid. In a blender, add all ingredients and process. Add more water as needed to achieve a thick, but pourable consistency. Garnish with the

red bell pepper strips and drizzle the two different colors of sauces below.

Red sauce	*Green sauce*
½ cup base	¼ cup base
¼ cup red bell pepper	Small handful fresh cilantro
1 tsp raw tahini	¼ tsp sea salt or to taste
½ tsp sea salt or to taste	

Combine ingredients for red sauce and green sauce separately in a blender and process until smooth.

Almond Mousse Stuffed Peppers

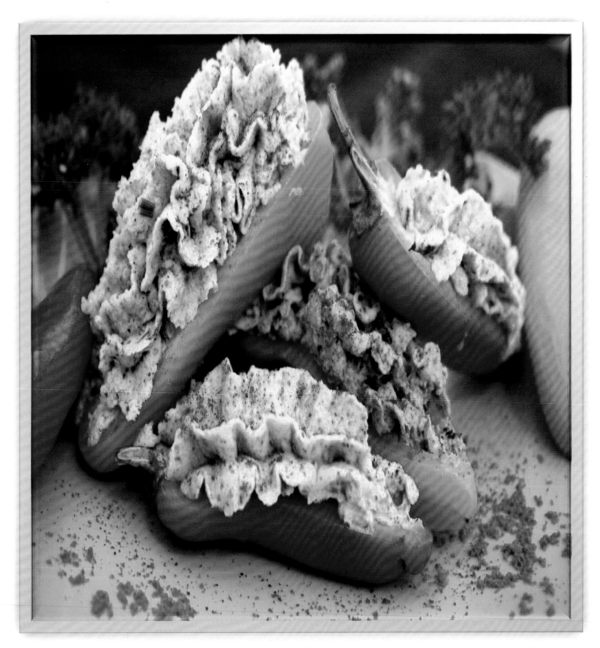

Almonds are a rich source of Vitamin E, containing 24 mg per 100 g. They are also rich in monounsaturated fat, one of the two "good" fats responsible for lowering LDL cholesterol. Experts discovered that almonds contain phenolics and flavonoids in their skins analogous to those of certain fruits and vegetables. For instance, a one-ounce helping of almonds holds a similar quantity of total polyphenol as ½ cup of cooked broccoli.

Almond Mousse Stuffed Peppers

3 ½ cups raw almonds

water

1-2 tsp sea salt

½ cup sundried tomato

¼ cup water

½ cup kalamata olives

2 Tbsp fresh flat leaf parsley

1 Tbsp fresh chive

¼ cup lemon juice

Cover almonds with the water by 2" and soak several hours or overnight.

In a sauce pot boil enough water to cover nuts to blanch them. This process will make it easier to peel off the skins. After water boils, add to nuts for about 5 minutes. Drain water and let nuts cool down. Pinch to remove skins.

Place the skinned almonds in a high speed blender. Add in the lemon juice, water, and salt. Process until smooth, using a pusher to help move the nuts around. It will be very thick.

Spoon half of the almond pate to a bowl, leaving the remaining half in the blender. To the blender, add the kalamata olives and chives and pulse until they are chopped fine.

Repeat with the other half of almond pate adding the sundried tomatoes and parsley. Each pate can be put into a piping bag and piped into hollowed-out peppers, as shown in the photo. Also try it piped atop thick slices of cucumbers. Use this for stuffing many other foods as well, as a spread, and as a dip. It is the most versatile mousse in raw foods.

Green Papaya Salad

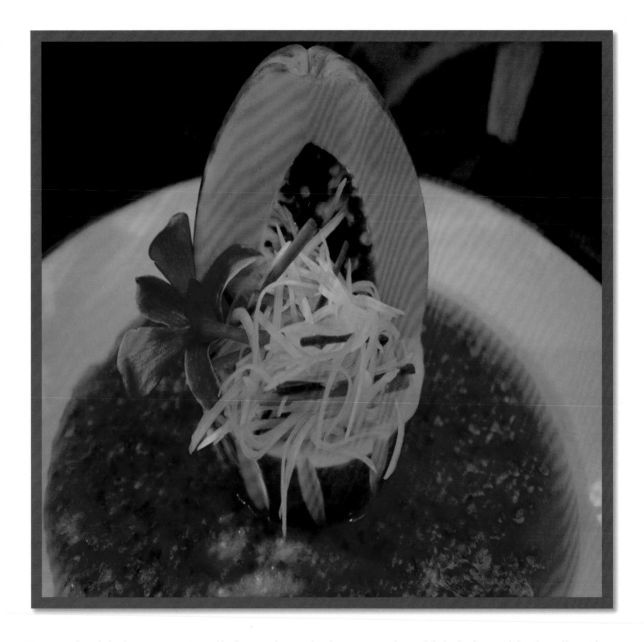

Papaya is rich in enzymes called papain and chymopapain which helps with the digestion, particularly it breaks down the proteins from the food we eat into amino acids. The latest research shows that amino acids are responsible for all what is happening in our organism, basically for what is happening in every chemical reaction as well as our mental and physical health.

Green Papaya Salad

2 med green papaya fine julienne

1 med carrot fine julienne

1 med cucumber skinned and fine julienne

chives opt. for garnish

Skin the papaya and rinse off sap.

Using a mandolin with a fine blade attachment, slice the papaya lengthwise into long strings, repeat with the cucumber and carrot. Place in a bowl and set aside.

Dressing—

1 large red bell pepper

1 Tbsp fresh mint leaves

½ cup olive oil

1 Tbsp fresh Thai basil

2 Tbsp lime juice

2 cloves of garlic

1 Tbsp agave

sea salt to taste

Cut off top with stem ½" deep. Cut off one wall of the pepper. This will result in a flat square of rectangle shape. Continue cutting each piece off, leaving the inner membrane and seeds intact with the bottom of the pepper. Place each piece flat with the skin down on the cutting board and with your knife parallel to the pepper, proceed to carefully and slowly slice the skin off the flesh as closely as possible. Repeat with the remaining peppers.

Place the bell peppers with the remaining ingredients in a blender and process until smooth. Adjust the salt to your taste.

Add dressing to strings and mix well. Let sit for an hour in the refrigerator to marinate. Serve on a lettuce leaf and garnish with mint and basil leaves, if desired.

Sprouted Bean salad

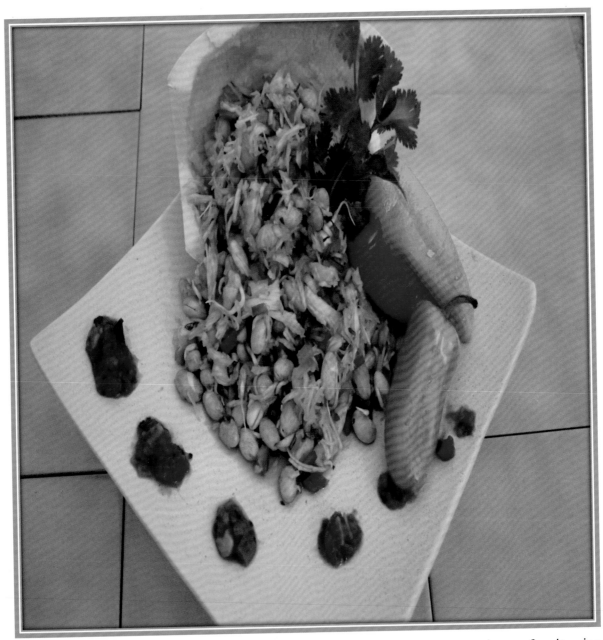

Sprouts are a great, inexpensive way of obtaining a concentration of vitamins, minerals and enzymes. They contain all of the nutrients found in the various fruits and vegetables. Eating sprouts is a safe way of getting the nutritional advantage of both fruits and vegetables without contamination and harmful insecticides.

Sprouted Bean salad

1 cup sprouted beans*

1 med spaghetti squash

½ red bell pepper small diced

½ cup green bell pepper small diced

¼ cup cilantro chopped fine

¼ cup green onion sliced fine

¼ tsp turmeric or mild curry powder

1 Tbsp elephant garlic minced

¼ Tbsp sea salt to taste

jalapeño to taste chopped fine

2 tsp flax seed oil

¼ tsp cumin

Rinse beans and soak overnight in 2-3 times the amount of water. Use a sprouting jar to rinse and store your sprouts. Rinse twice daily, each time draining the water and placing the jar upside-down in a darkened place. Do not place in cabinet or closet, it needs good circulation. After 3-5 days, depending on the type of beans you chose, your sprouts should be ready. Rinse and place in a container lined with paper towels. Store in the refrigerator until ready to use.

Cut squash down the middle remove seeds and pulp. Using a fork, gently scrape out the flesh. Place in large mixing bowl. Add the remaining ingredients and mix together. Let it sit for a few hours before served.

*Try sprouting adzuki, garbanzo, mung, or lentils. Be sure to use organic.

Nearly Raw Wrap

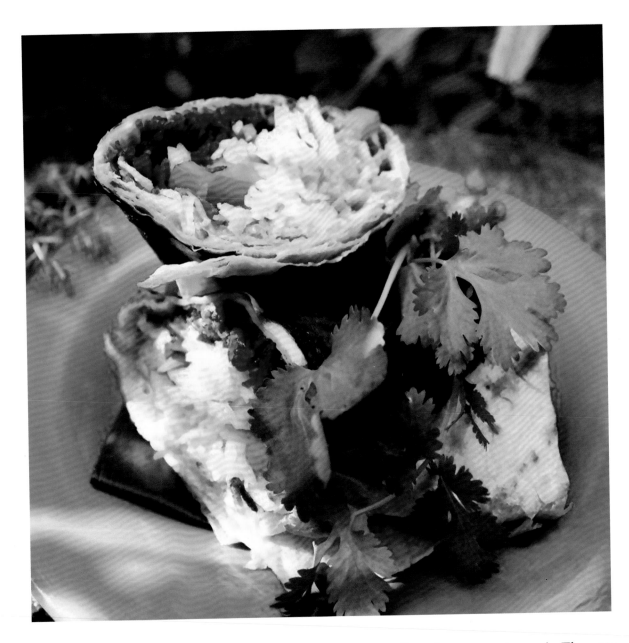

Raw foods are rich in enzymes. Enzymes are needed for the digestive system to work. They are necessary to break down food particles so they can be utilized for energy. The human body makes approximately 22 different digestive enzymes which are capable of digesting carbohydrates, protein and fats. Raw vegetables and raw fruit are rich sources of enzymes.

Nearly Raw Wrap

1 large carrot peeled

2 medium beets peeled

1 large cucumber–part of skin removed

½ Daikon radish peeled

1–bag seasoned corn chips (spicy)–crushed

5–sheet nori (dried seaweed or sushi)

1 large avocado

5 romaine leaves rinsed

5– 12'' tortilla wrappers

1 medium tomato

Plate of water

Use a mandolin to shred carrots, beets, cucumber, and radish into fine shreds. Finely slice tomato and avocado.

Warm tortilla wrapper by holding over the stove burner. Warm each side. Place the wrapper on a flat working surface. Layer the carrots, beets, cucumber, radish, tomato and avocado on the wrapper and sprinkle some crushed corn chips over. Top with the lettuce leaf. Roll by folding the left and right edges toward the center. Bring up the bottom and tuck with your fingers as you roll toward the top edge.

Dampen a sheet of nori in the water and quickly roll over the outside of tortilla wrapper.

Let stand for several minutes before slicing in half at an angle.

Napa Cabbage Kim Chee

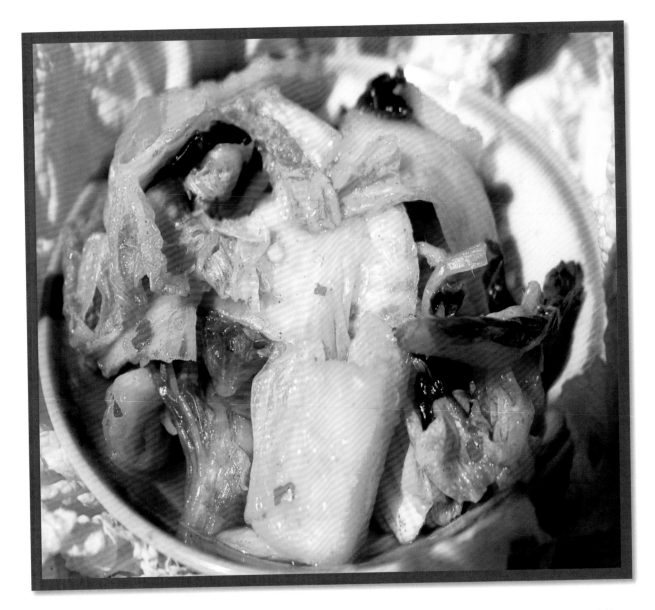

Kimchee is on the list of top five "World's Healthiest Foods" for being rich in vitamins, aiding digestion, and even possibly reducing cancer growth. However, some research focused on high-sodium dietary dependence has found overconsumption of kimchi and doenjang to be a risk factor in gastric cancer (most likely due to nitrates and salt) while unfermented alliiums and unfermented seafood were found to be protective factors. One oncological study found one type of kimchi to be a protective factor against gastric cancer while two other types of such high-sodium kimchi as dongchimi were risk factors.

Napa Cabbage Kim Chee

3 heads won bok (Chinese) or Napa cabbage

1 cup green onion chopped

¼ cup minced garlic

1 Tbsp minced fresh ginger

2/3 cup organic cane sugar

1/3 to ½ cup sea salt (depending on the size of the cabbage)

2/3 cup paprika

Dried chili pepper or Sambal Oelek hot sauce

Wash cabbage leaves and dry very well – cut into 2 inch sections, leaving just a small portion of the base. Discard the base. Place the chopped cabbage into plastic or non-porous wide mouth container with a tight lid.

Add the salt and mix it in with your hands to make certain the salt is evenly spread.

Find an area in your home with shade and somewhat cool. And place your container there; flip the container over every 8 hours, for the next two days.

On the second day, combine remaining ingredients in a processor and blend till smooth. Marinate this mixture for a few hours before adding to cabbage.

Stir the mixture into the cabbage. Do not discard the water from cabbage unless it is too salty, mix into the cabbage and liquid very well. Replace the lid.

Again, store in a shady spot for another day and resume flipping the container on the third day.

It should be ready on day four. Store in a covered container in the refrigerator up to two weeks.

Avocado Mousse

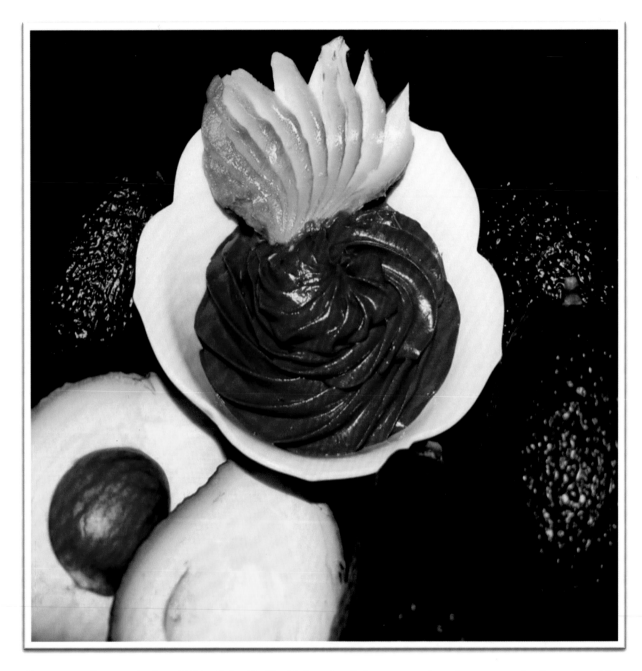

One cup of avocado has 23% of the Daily Value for folate, a nutrient important for heart health. Individuals who consume folate-rich diets have a much lower risk of cardiovascular disease or stroke than those who do not consume as much of this vital nutrient.

Avocado Mousse

2 large avocado

1/3 cup nut or rice milk

2 Tbsp carob powder

4 Tbsp agave or organic cane sugar

1 Tbsp yacon syrup

sea salt to taste

Combine all ingredients into high speed blender and blend till smooth.

Place into pastry bag and pipe out. Chill before serving.

Fast Foods

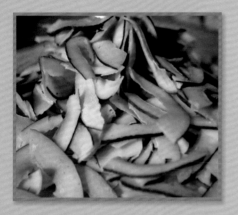

COCONUT CANDY

Take dried coconut, remove husk and drain water, cut white flesh out. Slice thin, using a mandoline if possible. Sprikle lightly with organic cane sugar. Place in oven at 170 degrees for 4-6 hours, or until nice and crispy-browned.

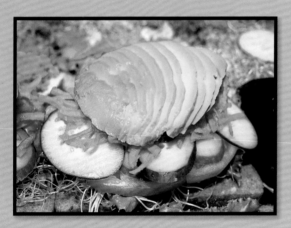

AVO-SANDWHICH

Whole wheat bread, Vegenaise, lettuce, sprouts, sliced tomato and cucumber, and shredded carrots.

Not only are avocados a rich source of monounsaturated fatty acids including oleic acid, which has recently been shown to offer significant protection against breast cancer, but it is also a very concentrated dietary source of the carotenoid lutein; it also contains measurable amounts of related carotenoids.

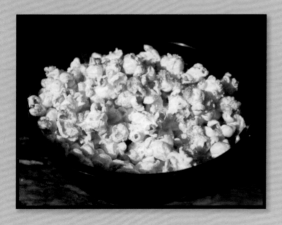

POPCORN

Air-popped popcorn, sea salt, nutritional yeast, olive oil, smoked paprika, garlic powder. All to taste

This can make it an attractive snack to people with dietary restrictions on the intake of calories, fat, and/or sodium.

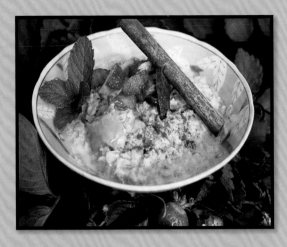

ROLLED OATS

2 parts water 1 part oats

Boil water, turn off heat, add oats wait for 10 minutes, and it's done.

Flavored with cinnamon, fresh strawberries, dates, maple butter and almond milk

Oats, via their high fiber content, are already known to help remove cholesterol from the digestive system that would otherwise end up in the bloodstream.

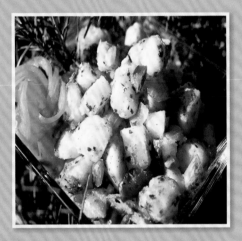

BREAKFAST –POTATO

Utilizing left over baked or roasted potatoes, they go well in the pan with:

onions, garlic, bell peppers, rosemary, and paprika.

Cook over medium-high heat and add some olive oil. Brown everything.

The results of a study suggest that carsnosic acid, found in rosemary, may shield the brain from free radicals, lowering the risk of strokes and neurodegenerative diseases.

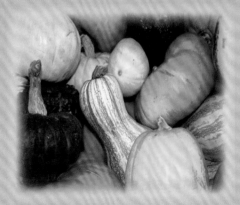

SQUASH

The quickest cooking method is to cut any squash in half, put into oven at 400-450 degrees till brown on top, then spoon and eat. Another way is cutting in bite size cubes, tossing with olive oil, fresh chopped herbs, and garlic- roast in the oven till brown, serve and eat- you can peel of the skin when you eat it—also makes a great soup this way.

It is a good source of fiber, vitamin C, manganese, magnesium, and potassium. It is also an excellent source of vitamin A.

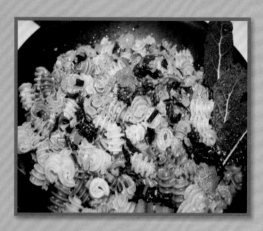

QUINOA PASTA

Cook pasta then set aside. In sauté pan, heat olive oil, chopped garlic, onions and fresh vegetables. I used fresh organic broccoli and kale. Sauté until tender then just add salt to taste. I like to use a lot of dark greens in my diet because of all the power it gives, but don't overcook them. You'll always want to add them last to cooked dishes. Try getting all organic when possible- going organic keeps the bitter pesticides off your plate and your pallet, making dark greens tasteful and healthful.

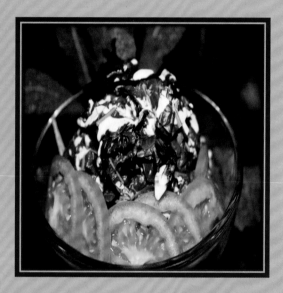

R-G-B   Rice, Greens, Bean

Cooked brown rice, cooked black beans, steamed chard or kale, fresh tomato, and flavored white sauce, from page-141.

This was a big seller on our trailer, so simple and so easy.

The vitamin K provided by Swiss chard in one cup of cooked Swiss chard, is important for maintaining bone health. Vitamin K1 helps prevent excessive activation of osteoclasts, the cells that break down bone.

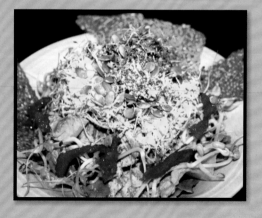

GREEN SALAD

Fast and easy, but what's on it makes the salad.

Pumpkin seeds-May promote prostate health, protection for men's bones, Anti-Inflammatory benefits in arthritis
Nutritional yeast-Some brands of nutritional yeast, though not all, are fortified with vitamin B12.
Chia seed-a super-nutritious superfood.
Flax seed- are rich in *alpha linolenic* , an omega-3 fat that is a precursor to the form of omega-3.

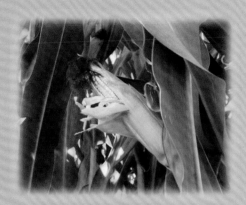

Corn on the Cob

We like it lightly steamed with fresh herbs. Basil, thyme, rosemary, oregano, and fresh garlic are put that into a food processor and chopped until fine. Add olive oil and infuse the oil in a pan over heat. Smear the corn in that oil and sprinkle with sea salt- great alternative to butter.

Corn as a good source of many nutrients including thiamin (vitamin B1), pantothenic acid (vitamin B5), folate, dietary fiber, vitamin C, phosphorus and manganese.

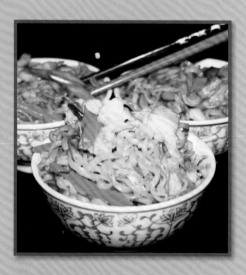

DRY MEIN

Use dry ramen or saimin noodles to make a great noodle dish. Here we have boiled the noodles until tender. Add garlic, fine chopped Napa cabbage, julienned carrots, and sliced green onions in a hot pan with sesame oil. Stir-fry everything. Add soy sauce to flavor. You can use any of your favorite dry noodles, and adding fresh vegetables to the noodle are a better meal for you, instead of using the dehydrated vegetable package that comes with it.

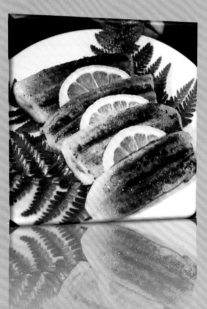

BROWN BANANA

This has got to be one of the best tasting and simple sweet. Take a firm, ripe banana and cut them into quarters. Use a non-stick skillet on medium high heat, adding just a few drops of oil, lay banana cut side down and brown. Sprinkle with cinnamon, nutmeg, and a pinch of salt. Turn over when brown, then reduce heat then sprinkle cinnamon sugar on other side. Turn off heat and leave fruit in pan till it's cooked all through. Squeeze lime or lemon juice over.

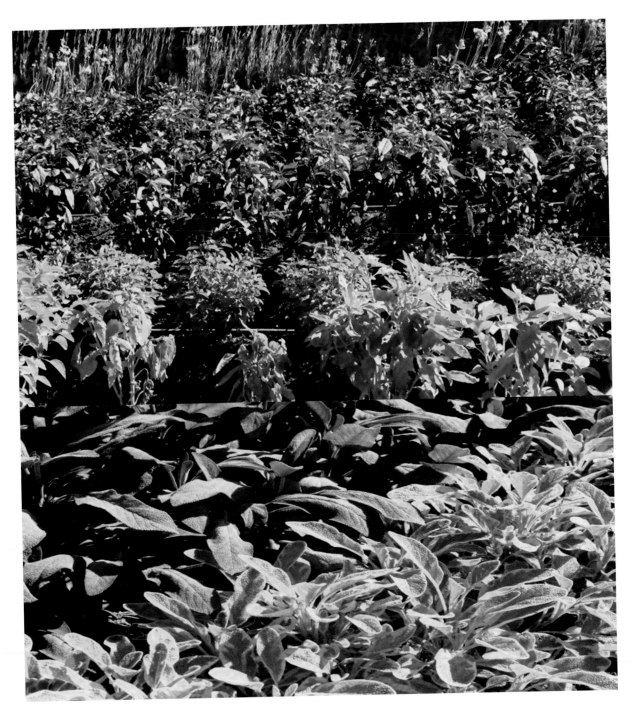

Herbs are not only aromatically fragrant but also contain tremendous healing capabilities. The botanical kingdom offers an enormous and exciting range of healing powers as well as breathtaking beauty. Prescriptive drugs are modeled after molecules found in nature

Entrees

Peperoni Di Polenta con la salsa Di Puttanesca

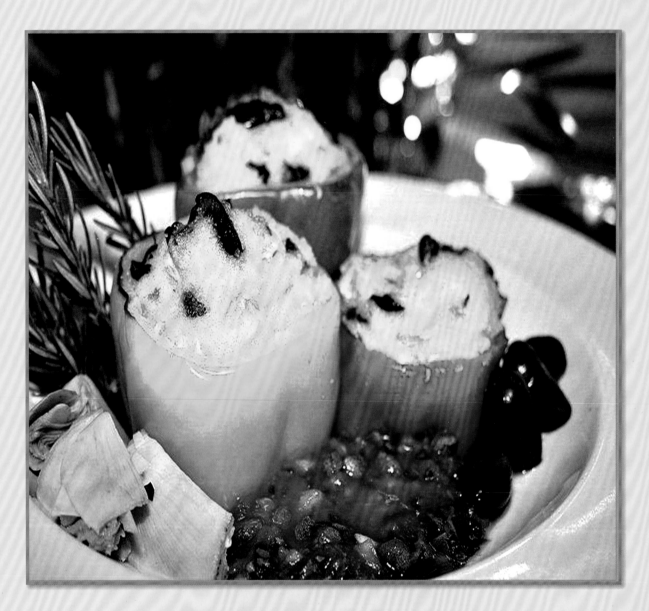

Polenta or "Italian grits" is the base for this dish called Puttanesca which originates in Naples. Like the meaning of the name, it's easy. Red bell peppers contain one of the highest concentrations of vitamin C and Kalamata Olives are very useful in helping relieve an upset stomach.

Peperoni Di Polenta con la salsa Di Puttanesca

4 red, green or yellow bell peppers

2 cups water

1 ½ cups coarse corn meal

½ onion chopped

¼ cup red bell pepper small dice

¼ cup green bell pepper small dice

1 Tbsp chopped garlic

1 Tbsp oil

½ Tbsp sea salt or to taste

3 Tbsp pitted Kalamata or black olives slivered

Rinse bell peppers and cut off top ½," leaving the stem intact. Scoop out seeds and large membrane. Set aside. In a small sauce pot, heat oil over medium-high heat. Add the onion, garlic and bell pepper and sauté for a few minutes. Pour in the water and add the salt—bring to boil. Next, add the cornmeal and cook until it is thickened. Remove from heat and stir in the olives. Use a spoon to stuff the hollowed-out bell peppers. Place in a baking dish and cover with foil. Bake at 350 degrees for 30 minutes until bell peppers are tender.

Puttanesca Sauce

3 Tbsp extra virgin olive oil

1 onion finely diced

½ green bell pepper finely diced

8 pieces Kalamata or black olives

1 Tbsp flat leaves parsley fine chopped

2 Tbsp capers

½ tsp sea salt

1 Tbsp garlic chopped

14 oz canned tomatoes

Crushed red pepper flakes

In a sauce pan, heat oil over medium-high heat, add the onion, garlic, green pepper. Sauté until browned. Add in the tomato and remaining ingredients. Reduce heat and simmer for 25 minutes. Add more salt if needed.

Portabella with Red Teriyaki Sauce

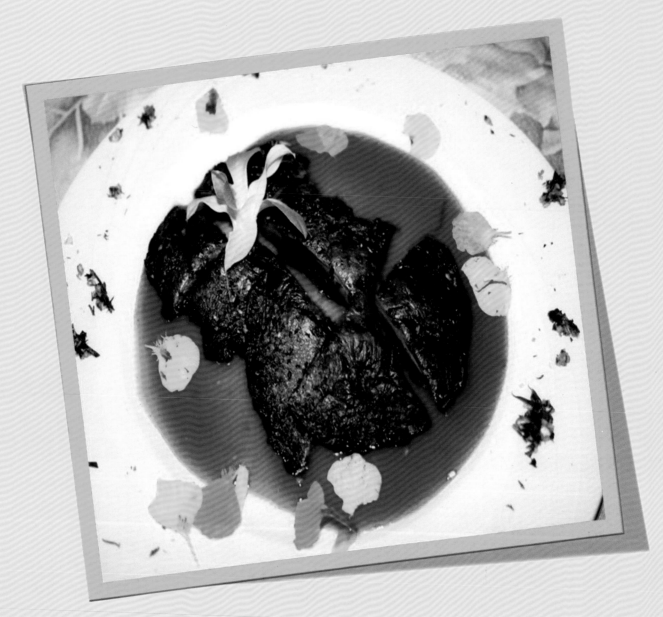

Portabella Mushrooms reign as the largest of the mushroom family growing up to six inches across. Their hearty texture makes them excellent in vegetarian meals. I suggest Portabellas smothered with olive oil, fresh garlic and herbs then grilled on an open fire.

Portabella with Red Teriyaki Sauce

4 large Portabella mushroom caps

¼ cup peeled garlic

1 Tbsp fresh rosemary

1 Tbsp fresh basil

1 Tbsp fresh thyme

½ cup olive oil

2 Tbsp lime juice

sea salt to taste

1 Tbsp fresh dill

Teriyaki Sauce p. 141

Marinara Sauce p. 143

Remove stems from mushrooms, rinse and pat dry. Set aside. Place garlic and fresh herbs in processor and chop till fine. Remove mixture and place in large mixing bowl with the olive oil and lime juice and let sit for 15 minutes.

Coat mushroom caps with oil and herb mixture and place on a barbeque grill. If a barbeque grill is not available then broil in the oven until browned and wilted, about 5–8 minutes. Sprinkle with salt and set aside to cool.

For the sauce, mix equal parts of Teriyaki Sauce and Marinara Sauce and warm in a saucepan over low heat.

Millet Sandwiches

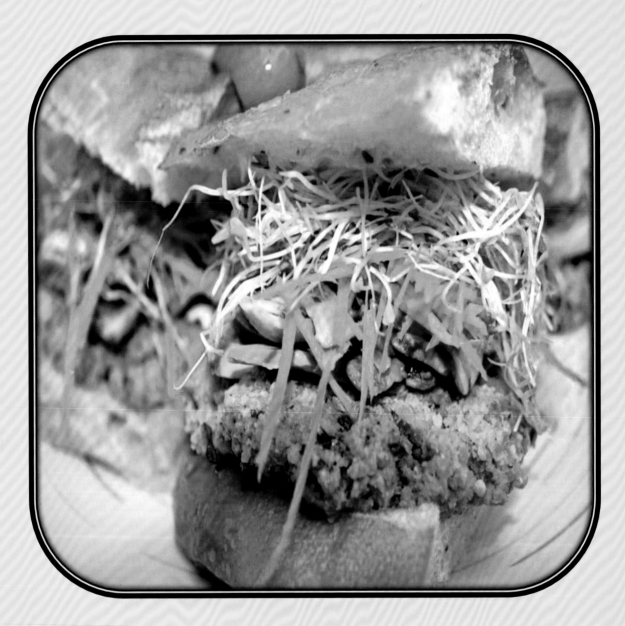

Scientific studies have established that compounds in basil oil have potent antioxidant, anti cancer, anti-viral, and anti-microbial properties. Traditionally used for supplementary treatment of stress, asthma and diabetes in India.

Millet Sandwiches

1 tsp olive oil

1 med onion small dice

5 cloves garlic small dice

1 rib of celery chopped fine

2 ½ cups water

¼ cup garbanzo bean flour

1 cup millet

1 tsp sea salt

1 tbsp fresh basil- fine chopped

1 tbsp fresh dill fine chopped

2 tbsp wheat germ

Heat the oil in a medium saucepan over medium-high heat. Add the onion, garlic and celery. Sauté until softened and browned. Add the water, millet and salt, bringing to a boil. Reduce heat and cover. Let simmer until liquid is absorbed and millet is soft. Allow to cool about 15 minutes.

Fold the basil, dill, wheat germ and garbanzo bean flour into the cooked millet. Use a 3oz. measure or portion scooper and form patties. Place the patties on an oiled sheet pan and bake at 350 degrees for 15-20 minutes or until lightly browned. Or drizzle olive oil in a sauté pan and brown on each side.

Shown in the photo: millet patties on toasted sourdough with avocado, grated fresh carrots, alfalfa sprouts, and sautéed garlic and mushrooms. Feel free to dress your sandwich as you choose.

Millet Patties with Tomato and Mushroom Sauce

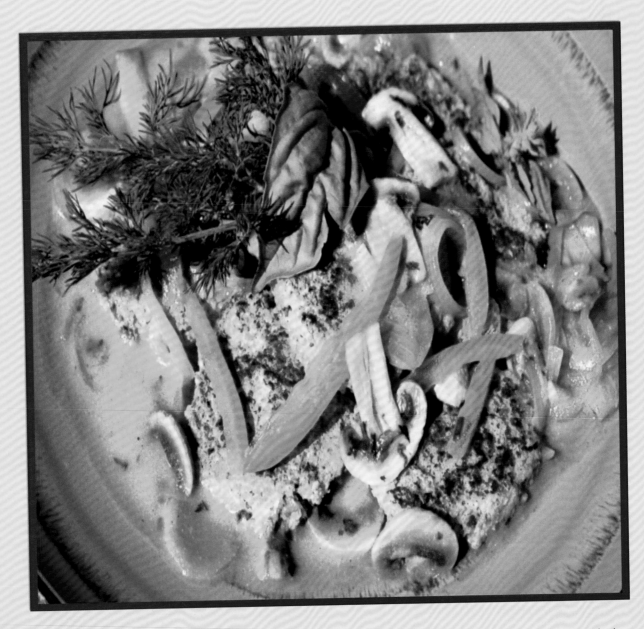

The protein content in millet is very close to that of wheat. Each provides about 11% protein by weight. Millet is rich in B-vitamins, especially niacin, B6 and folic acid. Also high in calcium,, iron, potassium, magnesium and zinc.

Millet Patties with Tomato and Mushroom Sauce

Sauce-

1 onion fine dice	2 tsp paprika
5 cloves garlic fine dice	1 tsp soy sauce
¼ cup light olive oil	2 cups water
¼ cup whole wheat flour	sea salt to taste
8 button mushrooms sliced	sliced tomato for garnish

Follow directions for Millet Patties on page 80. You may choose to omit the herbs.

Heat one tablespoon of the oil in a sauce pan over medium heat. Add the onion, garlic, and mushroom. Sauté until tender. Add the remaining oil. Stir in the flour using a wooden paddle, browning the flour for few minutes. Add the water, using a whisk to remove clumps and bring to a low boil, stirring often. Add the soy sauce and paprika. Season with salt to taste, adding more water as needed for desired consistency.

Garnish with a sliced tomato with the seeds and skin removed.

Farfallone e Porcini

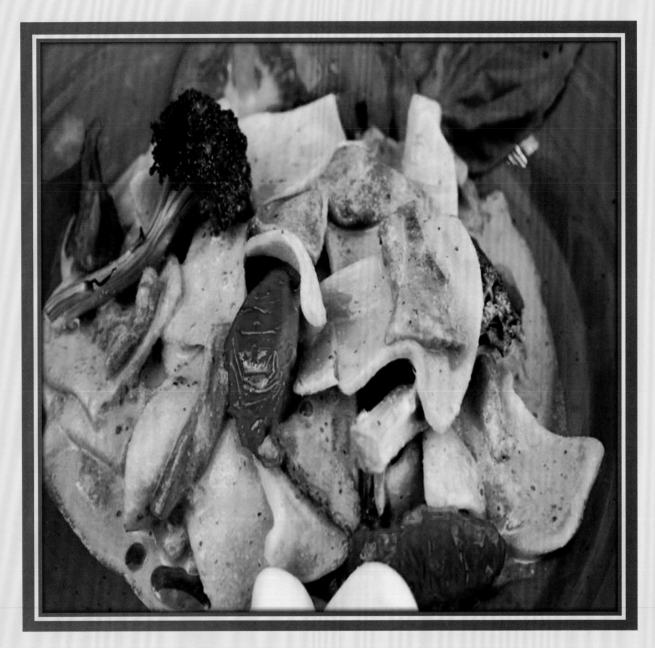

It is known as the Cep in France and Porcini in Italy. But here in the States, it is simply known as The King for it has become best loved for its firm texture and distinctive flavor.

Farfallone e Porcini

25 grams Porcini mushrooms, dried

4 cloves garlic sliced

½ white onion small dice

1 cup coconut milk

Sun dried tomato for garnish

1 tsp olive oil

1 lb cooked Farfallone (or other pasta)

2 heads broccoli

juice from 1 lemon

sea salt to taste

1 cup warm water

flax oil for drizzling

Soak mushrooms in 1 cup warm water until soft, set aside while preparing the noodles and sauce.

Remove crown from broccoli and cut into bite-sized pieces. Blanch the broccoli in boiling water until bright green and still firm, about 3 minutes. Toss with lemon juice and ½ tsp salt and lay on a baking sheet. Place the broccoli under the broiler or on grill to char. Set aside.

Cook pasta according to package directions. Drain and set aside.

Heat the oil in a sauce pot over medium heat. Add the onion and garlic. Sauté till tender.

To the sauce pot, add the soaked mushrooms along with the water. Increase the heat to medium-high and bring the mixture to a boil for two minutes. Stir in the coconut milk, returning the mixture to a boil for 5-10 minutes. This will reduce the sauce, making it thicker. Add salt to taste. Reduce heat to low.

Add the pasta to the sauce and toss gently. Gently stir in the broccoli and sun dried tomatoes and finish with a drizzle of flax oil. Serve immediately.

Au Gratin Potato with Red Bell Pepper Sauce

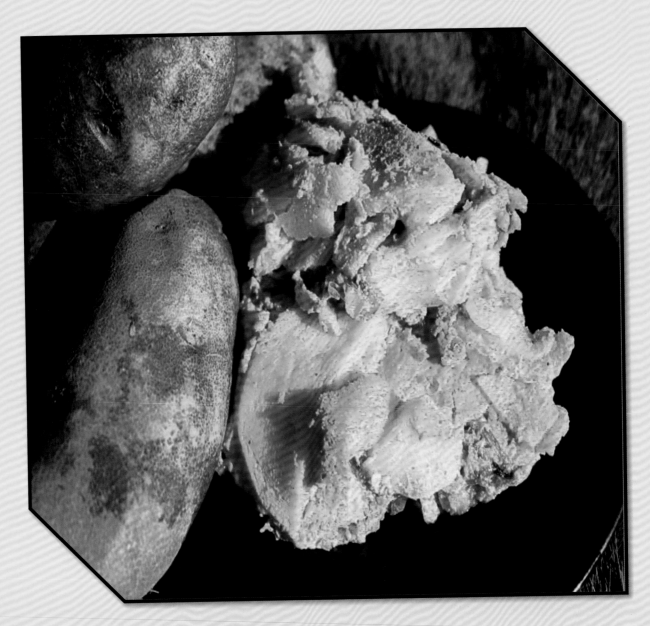

The fiber found in peppers can help to reduce the amount of contact that colon cells have with cancer-causing toxins found in certain foods or produced by certain gut bacteria. In addition, consumption of vitamin C, beta-carotene, and folic acid, all found in bell peppers, is associated with a significantly reduced risk of colon cancer.

Au Gratin Potato with Red Bell Pepper Sauce

7 large russet potato

½ large onion

½ roasted red bell pepper

½ cup raw cashews

6 cloves garlic

1 Tbsp olive oil

1 tsp sea salt or to taste

½ tsp nutmeg

½ tsp smoked paprika

1 ½ cup water

1 Tbsp lemon juice

2 Tbsp nutritional yeast

Pre-heat oven to 350 degrees.

Peel and slice potatoes 1/8" thick. Soak in cold water and set aside. Slice the onion thin and sauté in a pan with 1 tsp. olive oil until it is caramelized. In a 9" x 9" baking dish, place a third of the potatoes in a layer. Scatter half of the caramelized onions on top of that. Repeat with the second portion of potatoes and then the onions again. Add the remainder of potatoes for the last layer.

To the blender, add the red bell pepper, cashew, garlic, oil, salt, nutmeg, paprika, water, lemon juice and nutritional yeast. Blend until smooth. Pour the sauce over the potatoes. Place the dish on a sheet pan and cover with foil. Bake for 45-60 minutes or until potatoes are cooked through and sauce is thickened.

Veshable Mushroom

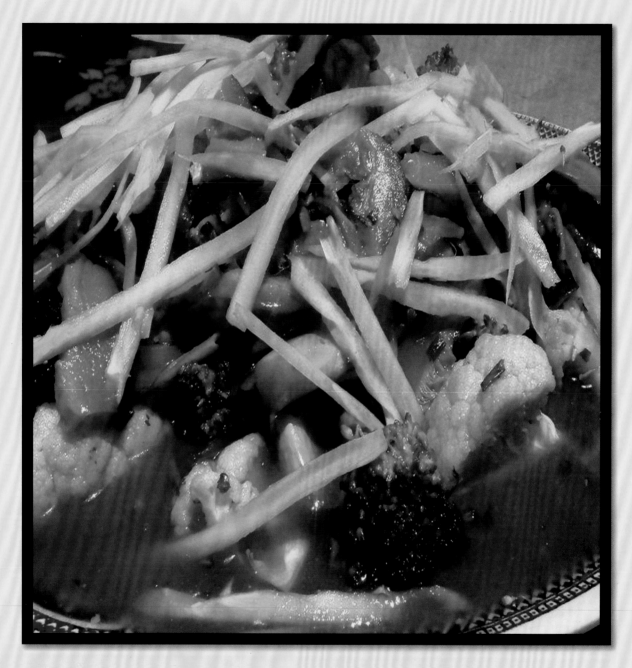

Shiitake Mushrooms have the ability to power up the immune system, strengthening its ability to fight infection, disease and powerful against influenza and other viruses.   Add this flavorful and unique healing food to many dishes

Veshable Mushroom

3/4 cup dried shiitake

2 large heads broccoli

1 large head cauliflower

1 Tbsp fine chop garlic

2 tsp fine chop ginger

2 Tbsp cornstarch in 2 Tbsp water

1 Tbsp sesame oil

1 ½ cup warm water

1 Tbsp fine chopped cilantro

3 Tbsp soy sauce

Soak mushrooms in warm water and set aside.

Rinse broccoli and cauliflower, remove stems and set aside. Cut the crowns into bite-sized pieces.

In a wok or a skillet, heat the pan over high heat and add the broccoli and cauliflower. Pour in the sesame oil (to keep it from burning) and use a wooden paddle to stir the vegetables around for about 2 minutes.   Add in the garlic, ginger and cilantro. At this point, cover with a lid to allow it to steam for a minute. Lift lid and add the mushrooms with water and continue to allow it to steam for another minute. Add the soy sauce and cornstarch/water mixture. Stir to thicken. Remove from pan onto a serving dish.

Peel hard skin from the stems of the broccoli and discard. Using a fine blade on a mandolin slicer, julienne the broccoli stem, creating fine shreds. Sprinkle over the hot vegetable dish.   Drizzle with hot chili oil or chili pepper sauce, if desired.

Layered Enchilada

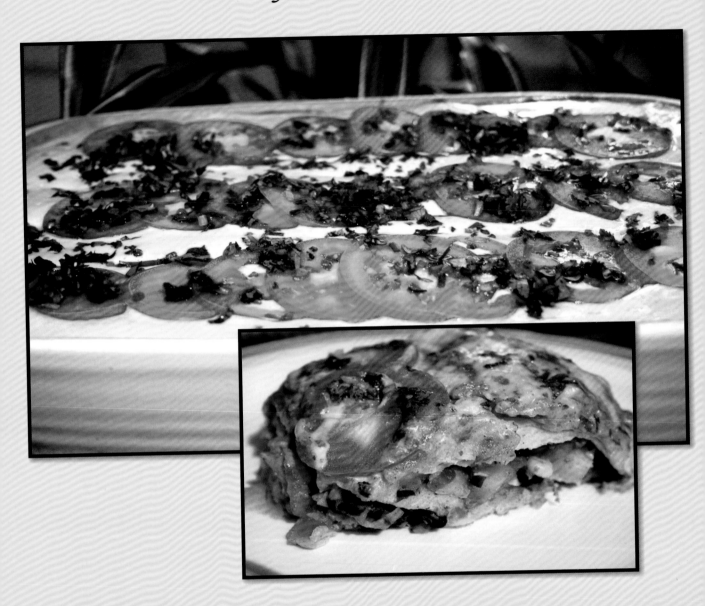

Layered Enchilada

1 med red onion small dice

2 large tomato small dice

1 cup corn kernels

½ cup cilantro, chopped

18- 6'' corn tortillas

1 green bell pepper small dice

2 large russet potato, peeled and small diced

½ cup green onion, chopped

8 oz black olives drained, small dice

Cook the peeled and diced potatoes in boiling water until just tender. Drain and let cool. In a medium bowl, combine the onion, tomato, corn, cilantro, green bell pepper, green onion, olives and cooled potatoes. Set aside. Soften the corn tortillas by heating individually in a pan or covered with a damp cloth and steamed, cut in half then set aside while preparing the Mole sauce.

Mole Sauce

4 each Ancho and New Mexico chile pods, stem and seeds removed then cover with hot water to soften.

6 cloves garlic

½ medium white onion diced

½ green bell pepper diced

2 Tbsp olive oil

½ tsp paprika

1 Tbsp curry powder

1 Tbsp cumin

1 Tbsp turmeric

2-3 Tbsp agave or organic cane sugar

½ tsp smoked paprika

¼ cup lime juice

1 tsp sea salt or to taste

Place softened peppers along with the water and garlic in a blender and process until smooth. In a saucepan, heat the oil over medium-high heat and add the onion and bell pepper. Sauté until softened and add the spices, stirring often for about half a minute. To this add mole sauce, lime juice and salt. Bring to boil. Reduce heat to low and simmer for 50 minutes.

Add 2 Tbsp cornstarch mixed with ¼ cup water to thicken. **You can also add 14oz. tomato sauce or 8 broiled Tomatillos.** In a casserole dish, layer with sauce, then corn tortilla, then filling, then sauce. Repeat layers, ending with sauce. Cover with foil and bake for 45 min at 350 degrees. Garnish with sliced tomatoes, cashew sauce or chopped green onions. Use extra mole sauce to serve on the side.

Spicy Eggplant

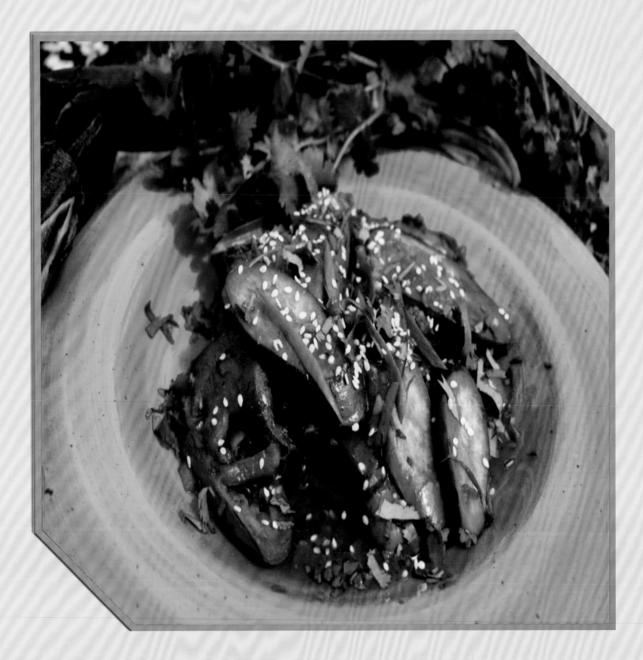

Salting and then rinsing the sliced eggplant is known as "degorging." This helps to soften and remove much of the bitterness though not always necessary. Some modern varieties do not need this treatment, as they are far less bitter. The nightshade is capable of absorbing large amounts of cooking fats and sauces, allowing for very rich dishes, but degorging will help to reduce the amount of oil absorbed.

Spicy Eggplant

2 Japanese eggplant

1 Tbsp chopped garlic

¼ cup sesame oil

1/8 tsp Indian Curry Powder p. 142

2 Tbsp plum sauce

1 Tbsp chopped cilantro

sesame seeds for garnish

1 Tbsp finely chopped ginger

1 Tbsp finely chopped lemon grass

½ cup Hoisin sauce

½ to 1 tsp Sambal Oelek (chili paste)

1 Tbsp chopped green onion

2 Tbsp soy sauce

Slice eggplant diagonally about ½" thick and place in a bowl. Sprinkle with salt on both side and let stand overnight. A brown liquid will appear. Rinse with water and drain well and pat dry with a paper towel.

In a small bowl, add the Hoisin and plum sauces together. To this mixture, add the garlic, ginger, lemongrass, curry powder, and Sambal Oelek and mix together, setting aside.

Heat the sesame oil in a sauté pan over medium-high and add the eggplant. Cook until browned and tender. Add in the sauce and reduce the heat to low, simmering and stirring occasionally. Add some soy sauce and adjust the salt as needed. Remove from heat then garnish with chopped green onion and/or cilantro and sesame seeds, if desired.

Rice Noodle Cake with Thai Sweet Sour Sauce

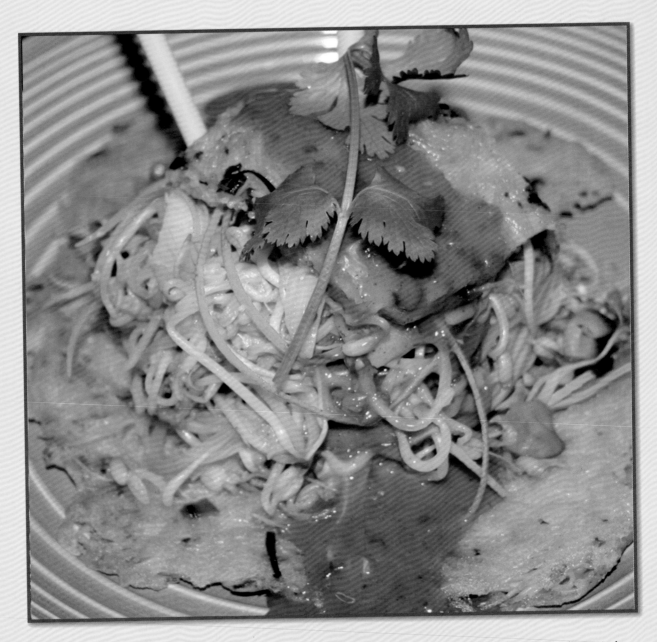

Tamarind is a good source of antioxidants that fight against cancer. Tamarind contains carotenes, vitamin C, flavanoids and the B-vitamins, reduces fevers and provides protection against colds helps the body digest food, is also used in treating bile disorders and can be gargled to ease sore throat.

Rice Noodle Cake with Thai Sweet Sour Sauce

Rice Noodle Cake

¼ cup olive oil

1 tsp turmeric

1 tsp paprika

2 cups cooked rice vermicelli

2 Tbsp green onion fine chopped

2 Tbsp cilantro fine chopped

sea salt to taste

Place the oil, turmeric and paprika in a small saucepan. Infuse the oil with the spices over low heat until. The oil will change become the color of the spices. Allow it to infuse for a few more minutes until the color becomes deeper. Strain the oil using a paper napkin or coffee filter.

Mix the vermicelli, green onions, cilantro and salt in a bowl. Add the infused oil to the noodles and mix well.

In a non-stick skillet heat a teaspoon of oil and place a handful of noodle mixture in the pan, flattening down to cover the surface of the pan. Brown for 3-5 minutes. Then turn over and brown for a few more minutes. Slice into various shapes, so it will sandwich the vegetables.

Stir-Fry Vegetables

1 carrot julienne

1 large cucumber julienne

 4 oz straw mushrooms

1 Tbsp sesame oil

1 cup chopped Napa cabbage

1 cup mung bean sprouts

1 Tbsp chopped garlic

In a wok or skillet, heat the oil and add the garlic, sauté till brown. Then add remaining vegetables, cook until tender. Remove from heat and place portions in between rice cakes. Drizzle sauce over the top.

Sauce-   In a sauce pan heat all the below ingredients until thickened.

½ cup coconut milk

1 tsp lemon juice

1 tsp tamarind paste

¼ tsp soy sauce

1/8 tsp paprika

1 tsp agave

¼ tsp pesto or Thai basil

1 tsp water mixed with 2 Tbsp cornstarch

Mixed Vegetables in Peanut Sauce

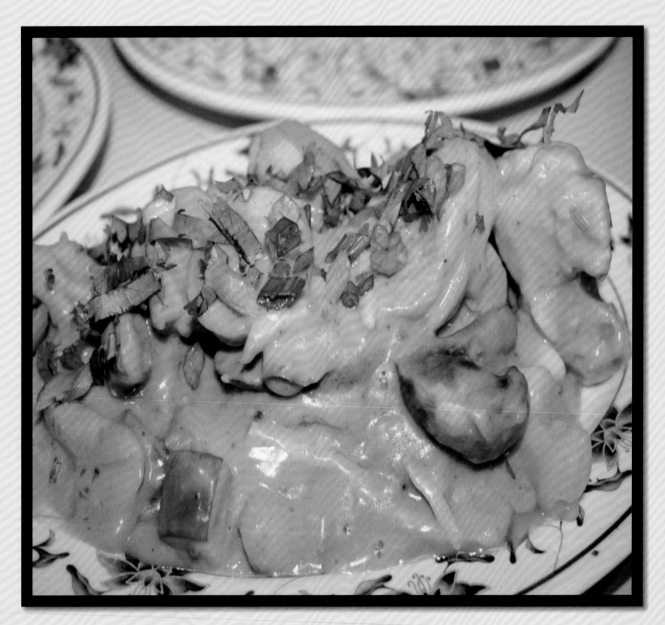

Peanuts are good sources of vitamin E, niacin, folate, protein and manganese. In addition, peanuts provide *resveratrol*, the phenolic antioxidant also found in red grapes and red wine. Not only do peanuts contain oleic acid, the healthful fat found in olive oil, but new research shows these tasty legumes are also as rich in antioxidants as many fruits.

Mixed Vegetables in Peanut Sauce

2 large carrots sliced on bias ¼" thick

1 large onion diced sliced

1 zucchini large diced

1 head of broccoli cut into bite-sized pieces

½ head cauliflower cut into bite-sized pieces

1 red bell pepper cut into large pieces

1 yellow squash large diced

2 potatoes large cubed

8 button mushrooms sliced

2 stalks green onion, chopped

2 Tbsp cilantro, chopped

Blanch the carrots, onion, zucchini, squash, cauliflower, bell pepper and broccoli in boiling water for 5 minutes. Remove the vegetables and place the potatoes, boiling until cooked and still firm. Cool with cold water and set aside.

Sauce

1 Tbsp sesame oil

1 Tbsp fine chopped ginger

1 Tbsp fine chopped garlic

15 oz coconut milk

7 oz creamy organic peanut butter

1/3 cup sweet Thai chili sauce

In sauce pan over medium-high heat, simmer the oil, ginger and garlic for two minutes to infuse the flavors. Pour in the coconut milk. Add the peanut butter and chili sauce and reduce heat to medium-low, allowing to simmer for 5 minutes.

Fold the prepared vegetables into the sauce. Garnish with cilantro and green onions.

String Patties with Chinese Douchi and Chili

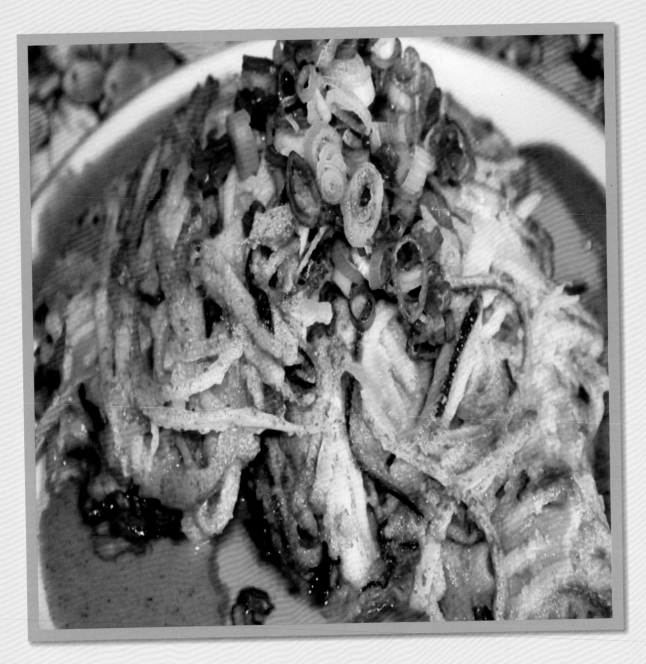

Douchi is made by fermenting and salting soybeans. The process turns the beans black, soft, and mostly dry. The flavor is sharp, pungent, and spicy in smell, with a taste that is salty and somewhat bitter and sweet.

String Patties with Chinese Douchi and Chili

1 carrot peeled and julienne very fine

2 zucchini julienne very fine

1 red bell pepper julienne very fine

1 medium onion sliced very fine

1½ cup garbanzo bean flour

1½ whole wheat flour

3 cups Water

olive oil for cooking

sea salt to taste

Mix the prepared vegetables together in a bowl. In a separate larger bowl, combine the flours and water and whisk together. The consistency should be thin. Drop in the vegetables and mix into batter very well.

In a non stick pan, add a tablespoon of oil and carefully drop in the battered vegetables, a half handful at a time, cooking until golden brown. Turnover and brown other side. Place on paper towels to absorb excess oil.

Sauce

Use White Sauce for base on page 141

1/2 cup base to 1 Tbsp douchi,

Sweet Thai chili sauce for a second sauce.

Spinach and Mushroom Buckwheat Crepes

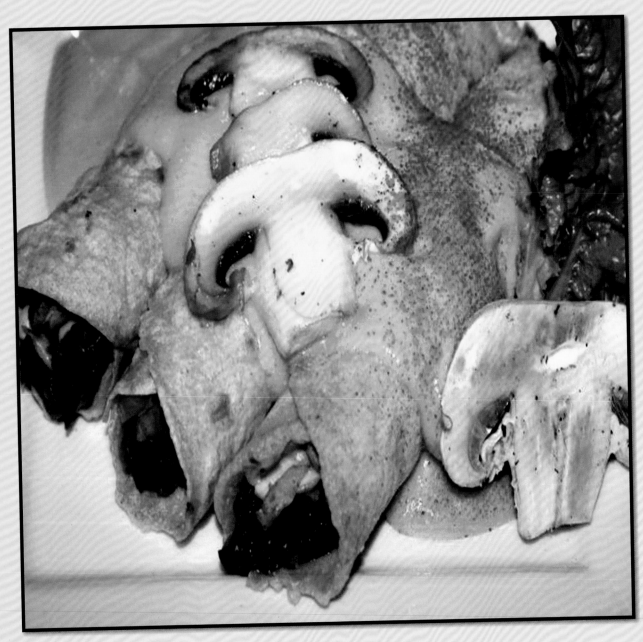

Spinach is an excellent source of vitamin K, vitamin A, manganese, folate, magnesium, iron, vitamin C, vitamin B2, calcium, potassium, and vitamin B6. It is a very good source of dietary fiber, copper, protein, phosphorus, zinc and vitamin E. In addition, it is a good source of omega-3 fatty acids, niacin and selenium.

Spinach and Mushroom Buckwheat Crepes

¾ cups raw cashews

3 cups water

1 cup raw potato, peeled and cubed

1 ½ cups buckwheat flour

1 cup unbleached flour

1 ½ tsp. sea salt

olive oil

Combine all ingredients in a blender and process until smooth. In a nonstick sauté pan, heat a teaspoon of oil over medium-high heat. Pour ¼ cup of batter into the pan and move the pan around so that the batter spreads evenly. Cook 1 minute then carefully slide onto a plate. Turn the plate over into the pan and brown the other side for 30 seconds.

Sauce:

1 cup raw cashews

1 – 15 oz can coconut milk

1 ½ tsp. sea salt

½ Tbsp lemon juice

2 tsp paprika

1 ½ cups water

3 Tbsp cornstarch

Combine all ingredients in a blender and process until smooth. Pour into a saucepan and allow it to thicken over medium heat, stirring with a whisk often to keep from scorching. When done, set aside.

Filling:

1 medium onion, chopped

3 cloves garlic, minced

8 oz. mushrooms, rinsed and sliced

2 zucchini, diced

olive oil

1 tsp sea salt

1 pkg. frozen spinach, thawed and excess water squeezed out

Sauté onion and garlic in 1 tablespoon oil till softened. Add in mushrooms and zucchini, season with salt, cooking until browned. Add in the spinach, stir to combine. Remove from heat and set mixture in strainer to drain excess liquid.

Roll filling in crepe and place seam side down in baking dish. Pour half the sauce over the crepes and cover with foil. Bake at 350 degrees for 25 minutes. Pour portions of remaining sauce onto plates and carefully place crepe on the sauce.

Whole Wheat Ravioli with Mushroom Duxelle

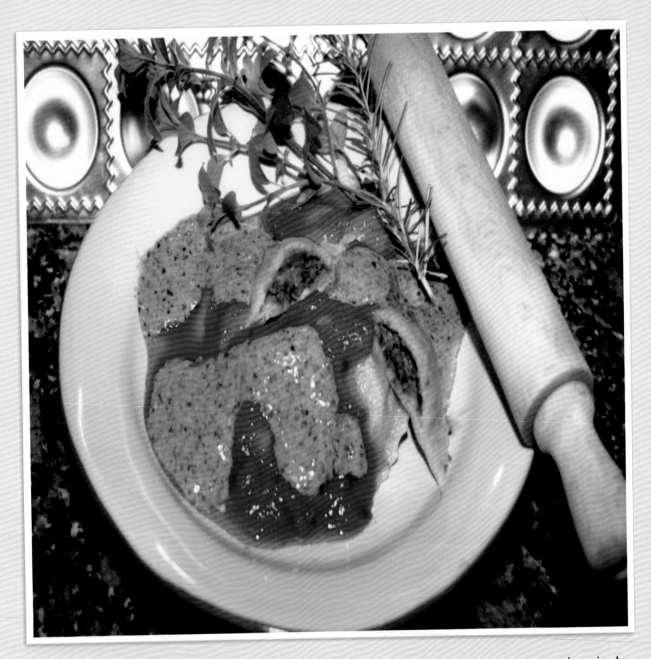

The white button mushroom has as much anti-oxidant properties as its more expensive rivals, the Maitake and the Matsutake mushrooms - both of which are highly prized in Japanese cuisine for their reputed health properties including lowering blood pressure and their alleged ability to fight cancer.

Whole Wheat Ravioli with Mushroom Duxelle

Dough

1 cup whole wheat flour

1 tsp sea salt

1 tsp oil

¼ cup water

Mix all ingredients to form dough. Shape into a ball and chill 20 minutes before using.

Duxelle

½ onion

1 Tbsp garlic

15 –18 button mushrooms rough cut

2 Tbsp olive oil

10 oz spinach

sea salt

Place onion, garlic, and mushrooms in a food processor and pulverize.

Using a non stick skillet, heat pan over high heat and add oil. Add the mushroom mixture, stirring often. Gradually reduce the heat as the liquid is being cooked out. This process may take up to 20 minutes.

About half way through cooking the above mixture, add spinach and continue cooking out the liquid. Stir often. Set aside and cool.

Remove dough from refrigerator and cut in half. Roll out one half to form thin sheets. Lay sheets out on a flat surface and place 1 ounce size potions evenly spaced apart about 1 ½". Roll out other portion of dough and cover the first sheet with the mounds of filling on it. Press to seal around the edges of each mound then use a cookie cutter to cut into individual ravioli.

Boil in water for 5-8 minutes until ravioli float to the surface. Cooking time will depend on how thick dough is. Serve immediately. The above picture is shown with a basil cream and a spicy marinara sauce. See recipe on pages 141,143.

Black Bean Tamales

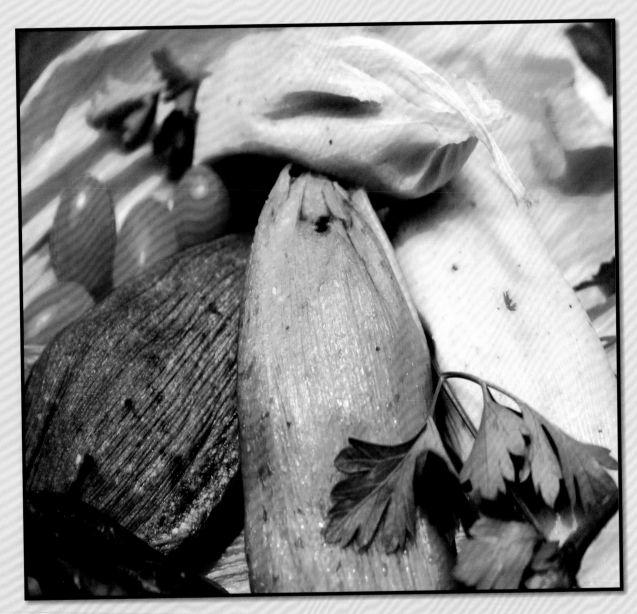

Charcoal was consumed in the past as dietary supplement for gastric problems in the form of charcoal biscuits. Now it is available in tablet, capsule or powder form and still used for digestive benefits. Charcoal absorbs gases and toxins to help heartburn, flatulence or indigestion. Charcoal is often used to filter water to remove bacteria and undesired tastes. In certain industrial process, such as the purification of sucrose from cane sugar, impurities cause an undesirable color, which can be removed with activated charcoal.

Black Bean Tamales

Filling

1 onion, chopped

1 green bell pepper, chopped

5 cloves garlic, minced

1 small bunch cilantro, chopped

2 Tbsp olive oil

1 Tbsp cumin

4-5 dried chile pods, remove stem and seeds, soak in hot water

1 ½ tsp sea salt

1 can black beans, drained

1 can corn

olives, chopped

2 zucchini, diced

any other vegetables as desired

4 oz tomato sauce

1 tsp dried or 1 Tbsp fresh oregano

Sauté vegetables in olive oil until softened. Add in the cumin and sauté for another minute. Add the chile pods which have been blended with the soak water. Add the beans, corn, tomato sauce and salt. Stir till combined and reduce heat to a simmer. Simmer until most of the liquid has been absorbed.

Masa

½ bag masa harina

1 cup olive oil

1 Tbsp sea salt

2 Tbsp. cumin

1 Tbsp. dried or fresh chopped oregano

6 chile pods, stem and seeds removed

7 cups water

1 pkg corn husk soaked in warm water

Cover the chile pods with hot water and soak until softened. Blend until smooth. Pour masa into a large bowl and add the chile puree, salt, oregano, cumin and olive oil. Gradually pour in half the water and mix. Continue to add more water until the consistency is spongy, almost sticky. If it is too dry, your final product will be hard, so add water as needed. Place about ½ cup masa on soaked and softened corn husk and 2 Tbsp filling. Wrap and steam for one hour. Tamales freeze well.

Mexican Pizza

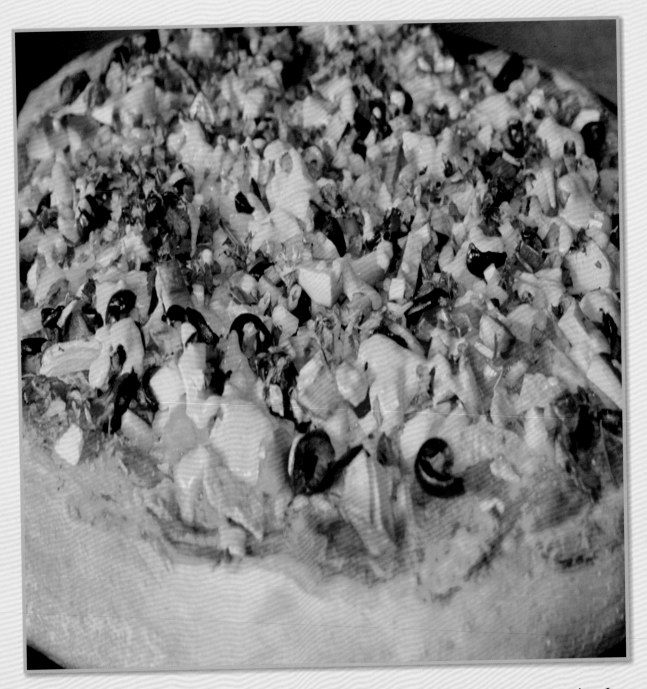

This is one of the pizzas I came up with when I use to work at the hotel in the pizza station. It was one of those pizzas you make only for special people.

Mexican Pizza

Dough

3.5 lb flour—any type of flour can be used

1 Tbsp sea salt

2 cups warm water about 120 degrees

½ cup organic cane sugar

3 Tbsp yeast

Combine all ingredients and knead for 15 minutes, then let stand for 45 or till risen, then punch down and roll out with a rolling pin or stretch by hand.

This makes 2 large pizzas

3 Tbsp Marinara Sauce p. 143

White Sauce p. 141

garlic powder

cumin

chili powder

turmeric

paprika

1 avocado sliced

black olives sliced

corn tortilla chips

tomato salsa

green onions chopped

cilantro chopped

Onto the prepared dough, spread the marinara sauce evenly. Sprinkle the garlic powder, cumin, curry powder and chili powder. Alternately, you many just use mole sauce. Over this, drizzle the white sauce.

Add the toppings in this order: crushed corn tortilla chips, tomato salsa (liquid drained), black olives, avocado, cilantro and green onions.

To 2 tablespoons of the white sauce, add a dash of turmeric and paprika. Mix well. Drizzle over the pizza last. Bake at 400 degrees for 15-20 minutes. Use either a pizza stone for a nice crust. Or use a pan coated heavily with olive oil and cornmeal sprinkled on.

Steam Baby Bok Choy with Colored Rice

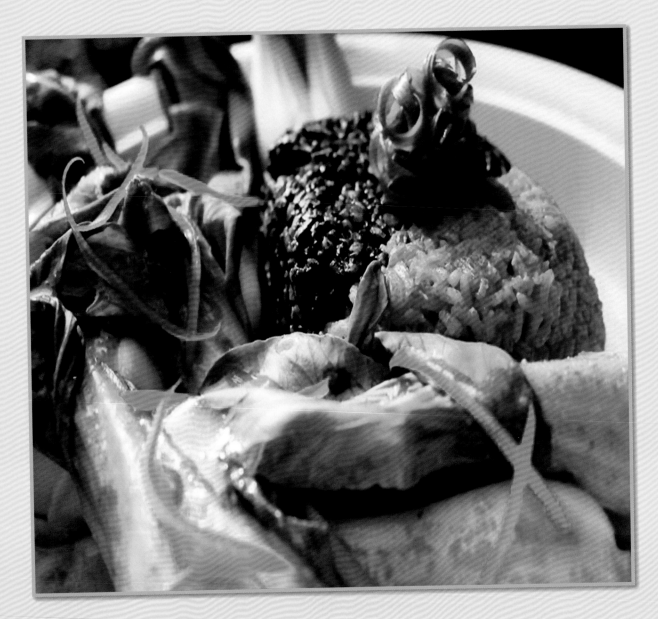

Bok Choy is high in Vitamin A, Vitamin C and calcium, but it is low in calories. Because both Bok Choy's stalks and leaves can be used in salads, it also provides a delicious and healthy meal for those who are on a diet. Bok Choy is also easy to prepare. You need only rinse it, chop it, then use it as you desire; for example, you can microwave or steam it for a simple and quick side dish or main meal.

Steam Baby Bok Choy with Colored Rice

6 baby Bok Choy – rinsed and cut in half

1 tsp fresh ginger

1 tsp garlic

¼ cup sesame oil

1 Tbsp tahini

½ tsp seasoned seaweed paste

1/3 cup olive oil

1 Tbsp soy sauce

1 tsp sesame seeds

2 Tbsp lemon juice

2 Tbsp agave or raw organic sugar

Steam the Bok Choy and set aside. Blend the remaining ingredients to make dressing and drizzle over or use as a dip.

Red rice

1 Tbsp olive oil

½ cup long grain brown basmati rice

½ cup onion

1 tsp paprika

1 rib of celery

½ cup water

2 Tbsp green bell pepper

sea salt to taste

Heat oil in sauce pan over high heat. Add the onion, pepper, and celery. Sauté for three minutes, then add paprika and rice. Coat the rice in the oil mixture and add water. Bring to a boil, then immediately reduce heat to low and cover. Simmer until rice is cooked.

Black rice

½ cup long grain basmati rice

1 ½ cups water

1 tsp charcoal powder

sea salt to taste

In a sauce pan add all ingredients, bringing to boil. Immediately reduce heat to low and cover. Simmer until rice is cooked.

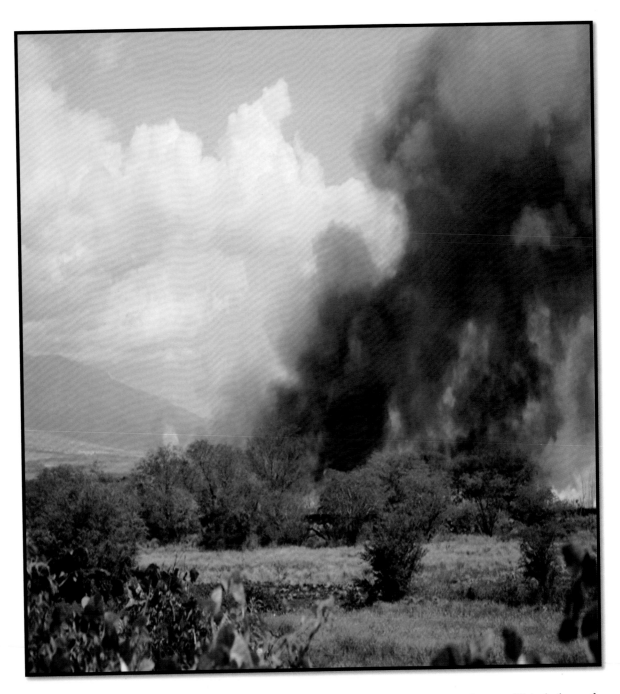

No, this is not a brush fire, but a real cane fire less than a mile from my home. This is how the sugar company cleans away most of the debris that is in the cane field. Not to mention all the pesticides and plastic that also goes up in flames, seeing one of these at night is quite impressive, unfortunately it's part of the process how we get our sugar.

Sweets

Ono Banana Bread

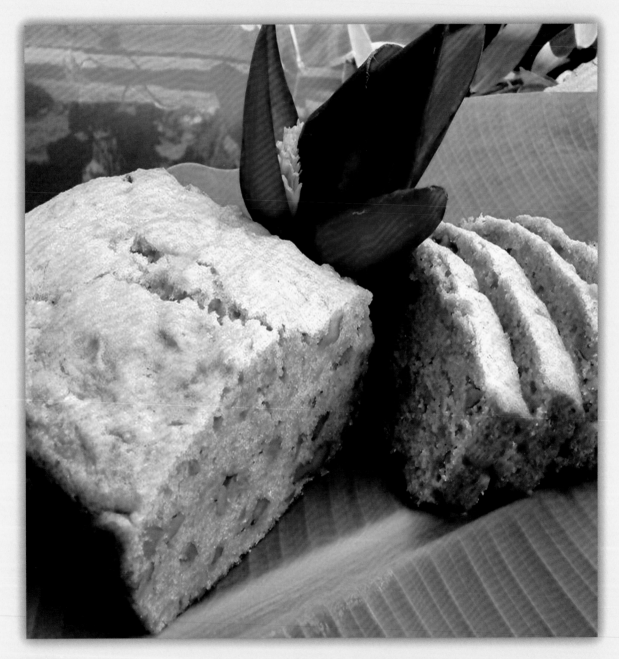

Bananas are one of our best sources of potassium, an essential mineral for maintaining normal blood pressure and heart function. Since the average banana contains a whopping 467 mg of potassium and only 1 mg of sodium, a banana a day may help to prevent high blood pressure and protect against atherosclerosis.

Ono Banana Bread

1 cup palm shortening

1 cup organic cane sugar

1 cup sucanat

1 tsp sea salt

4 cups mashed ripe bananas

2 ½ cups whole wheat flour

2 cups whole wheat pastry flour

2 cups chopped walnuts

1 Tbsp baking powder

Cream shortening, sugar and sucanat. Add the salt and bananas. Add flours, one cup at a time.
Fold in the walnuts and baking powder and stir to combine. Immediately pour into 3 oiled loaf pans
and bake in preheated oven at 350 degrees for 45-50 minutes.

Carob Cake with Ganache Frosting

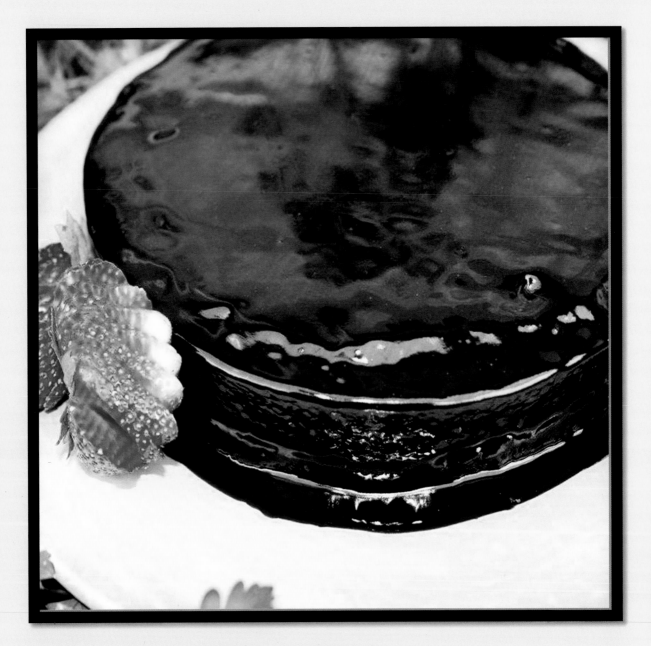

Virtually fat-free, is rich in pectin, is not allergenic, has abundant protein, and has no oxalic acid, which interferes with absorption of calcium. Consequently, carob flour is widely used in health foods for chocolate-like flavoring.

Carob Cake with Ganache Frosting

Carob cake

1 cup whole wheat flour, sifted

½ cup whole wheat pastry flour, sifted

¾ cup organic cane sugar

½ cup carob powder

¼ tsp salt

1 vanilla bean, scrape seeds

1 ½ tsp baking powder

¼ cup palm shortening

1 ½ tsp egg replacer mixed with 2 Tbsp water

¼ tsp almond extract

1 cup nut milk

Preheat oven to 350 degrees. Oil and flour an 8" round cake pan. (For a double-layer cake, make two recipes). In a bowl, combine the flours, sugar, salt and baking powder. Cut in the palm shortening.   In a small bowl, combine the egg replacer, lemon juice, almond extract, vanilla bean seeds, and milk. Add the liquid ingredients to the dry and mix well or use a hand blender to achieve a smooth consistency. Pour into prepared cake pan and bake 35-40 minutes or until knife inserted near the center comes out clean. Allow to cool completely on wire rack before frosting.

Carob Ganache

4 cups vegan carob chips

1 cup nut milk

1 Tbsp. brewed coffee substitute or 1 1/2 tsp. coffee sub. and 1/4 cup granules

1/4 cup maple syrup or agave

Place ingredients in the top of a double boiler. Heat until chips are melted, using a whisk to stir ingredients together. Set aside to cool. Refrigerate and warm slightly before frosting cake.

Poached Pair in Spiced Agave

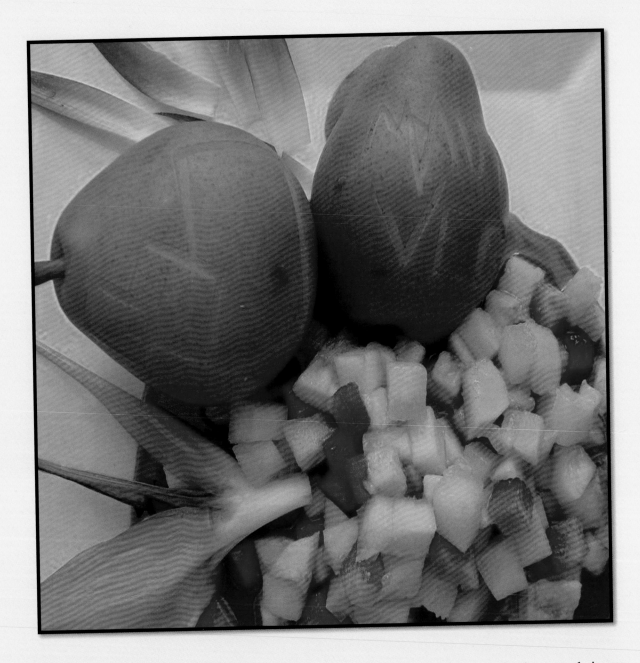

Pears are a good source of vitamin C, an important antioxidant necessary for bone and tissue health, and prevention of cardiovascular disease and various cancers. Pears are also a natural source of other antioxidants.

Poached Pear in Spiced Agave

Pear stock

2 pears

1 quart water

½ tsp ground ginger

2 cinnamon sticks

1 pinch salt

½ organic cane sugar

Agave sauce

1/3 cup agave

1 Tbsp ground coriander

1/3 cup coconut syrup

1 Tbsp brown sugar

1 Tbsp molasses

¼ tsp cinnamon

1 Tbsp yacon syrup

In a medium sauce pot, add water with the remaining ingredients and place pears in. Use a heavy ceramic plate on the pears to submerge them for even cooking. Bring to boil, and then reduce heat to low and simmer for 5-10 minutes until tender. At this point you can choose to have it cool or warm.

For the agave sauce: Put all ingredients into a small saucepan over low heat. Mix together until sugar dissolves. Use as a sauce or dip.

To chill the pears, cool down stock liquid and place pears back into it. Store in the refrigerator. To serve: Peel the pears, slice into halves or quartered and remove core with a melon ball scooper. Place arranged fruit on a plate drizzled with the agave sauce, garnish, and drizzle with more agave sauce on top. Serve.

Pineapple and Carob Spelt Muffins

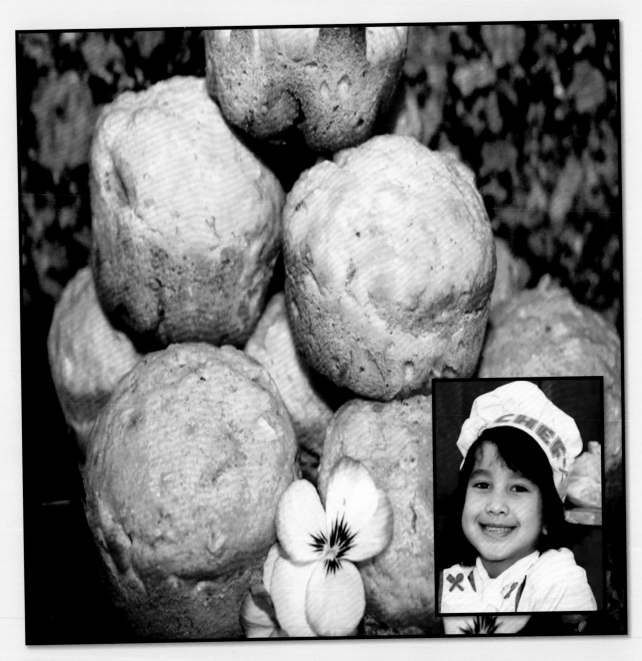

Spelt features a host of different nutrients. It is an excellent source of vitamin B2, a very good source of manganese, and a good source of niacin, thiamin, and copper. This particular combination of nutrients provided by spelt may make it a particularly helpful food for persons with migraine headache, atherosclerosis, or diabetes. My 8 year old daughter made these for me.

Pineapple and Carob Spelt Muffins

1 cup unbleached all purpose flour

½ cup spelt flour

½ cup millet flour

1 ½ tsp baking powder

½ cup organic cane sugar

½ tsp sea salt

¼ tsp cardamom

2 tsp olive oil

2/3 cup milk

1 Tbsp vanilla extract

1 cup canned pineapple + ½ cup liquid

½ cup apple sauce

½ cup slivered almonds

½ cup carob chips

Preheat oven to 350 degrees.

Combine the flours, baking powder, sugar, salt and cardamom. Use a wire strainer to sift all dry ingredients into a mixing bowl. Add the oil, milk and vanilla extract, apple sauce, mix to incorporate wet and dry ingredients, do not over mix. Fold in the fruits, almonds and carob chips. Pour batter into lined or oiled muffin pans and bake for 20-25 minutes or until toothpick inserted near center comes out clean.

Banana Bread Napoleon with Hazelnut Mango Sauce

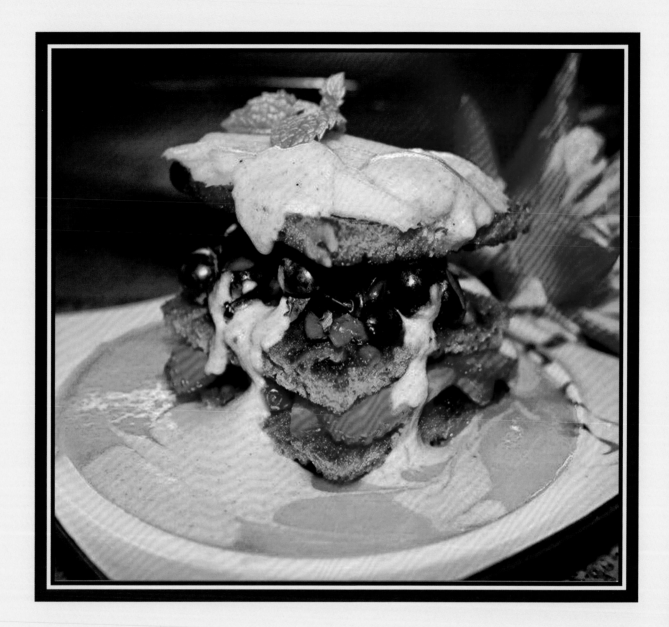

One cup of blueberries offers amount of vitamin C, minerals and phytochemical for only 83 calories. The pigments that give berries their beautiful blue and red hues are also good for your health. Berries contain phytochemicals and flavanoids that may help to prevent some forms of cancer.

Banana Bread Napoleon with Hazelnut Mango Sauce

3 slices mango bread ¼ inch thick p. 112

1 Tbsp walnut oil

½ cup hazelnuts or filberts

2 cups nut milk

1 Tbsp vanilla extract

¼ cup wheat germ

3 tbsp liquid sweetener or to taste

1 cup sliced fresh fruit

½ cup mango or fruit puree

Using a spray bottle, spray bread slices with oil and toast till crispy. This can be achieved by using a skillet or broiler. Then set aside after browned.

In a blender, add the milk and nuts, blending until smooth. Add the vanilla, wheat germ, and your choice of sweetener, blend.

On a serving dish, lay a slice of the toasted mango bread. On that, spoon a portion of the fruits. Repeat the layers and end with the mango bread. Pour the sauce over top and garnish with the fruit puree and a few more pieces of fruit.

Fool-Proof Whole Wheat Bread

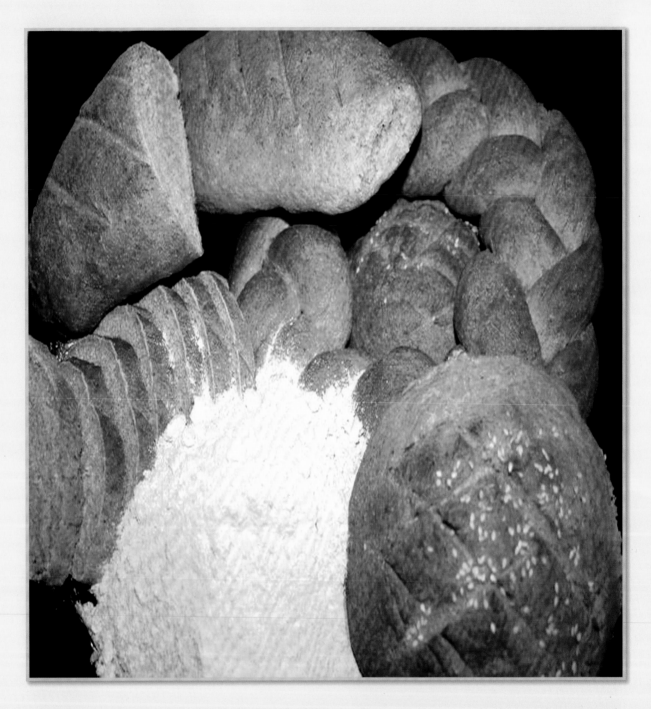

And Jesus said unto them, I am the bread of life: he that cometh to me shall never hunger; and he that believeth on me shall never thirst.   It's pretty hard to top that, in reference to bread.

Fool-Proof Whole Wheat Bread

3 lbs whole wheat flour

4 lbs unbleached flour

5 Tbsp yeast

2 Tbsp sea salt

1 cup organic cane sugar

2 quart water @ 120 degrees

Pre heat oven to 350 degrees.

To a large mixing bowl, add flours, yeast, salt and sugar and mix. Add the warm water slowly while continuing to mix. When the dough becomes too stiff to mix with a spoon, use your hands and knead the dough for 15 minutes. Cover with a clean towel and let rise for 45 minutes in a warm place. Punch the dough down and roll out into the desired shape and place on an oiled baking sheet. Allow to rise one more, 45 minutes. Bake for 30 minutes or until golden brown and a hollow sound is produced when tapped on. Rotate the sheet half way through baking.

We have done this bread by hand and machine and have used the same recipe with countless flavors, from sweet breads to herbs and garlic. Just add your extra ingredient after the water goes in. Then continue as directed.

Coconut Carob Pudding

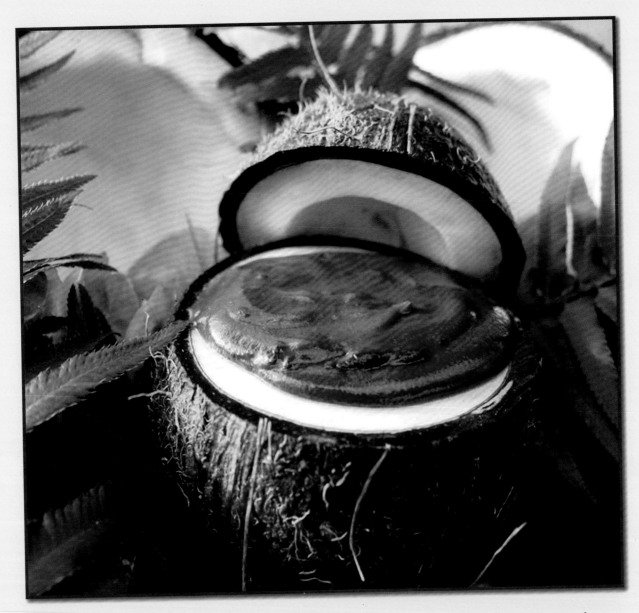

Coconut oil has been described as "the healthiest oil on earth, It is now gaining long overdue recognition as a nutritious health food. While coconut possesses many health benefits due to its fiber and nutritional content, it's the oil that makes it a truly remarkable food and medicine. Wherever the coconut palm grows the people have learned of its importance as an effective medicine. For thousands of year's coconut products have held a respected and valuable place in local folk medicine and now science is confirming its intrinsic values.

Coconut Carob Pudding

2 cups coconut milk

1/3 cup organic cane sugar or agave

1 Tbsp molasses

2 Tbsp cornstarch and water

½ water

1/3 cup yacon syrup

2 pinches sea salt

In a medium sauce pan combine all ingredients except cornstarch, mix well and place on medium low heat.

As the mixture starts to bubble rapidly, pour in cornstarch and using a whisk keep mixing to prevent from burning. Cook for another few minutes then portion out and serve either hot or chilled.

Makes 4 rich servings

Pumpkin Scones

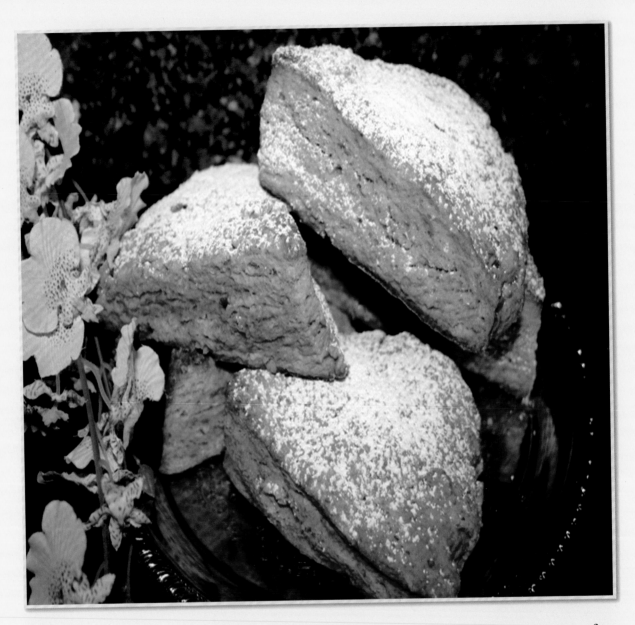

Pumpkin is very rich in carotenoids, which is known for keeping the immune system of an individual strong and healthy. Beta-carotene, also found in pumpkins, is a powerful antioxidant as well as an anti-inflammatory agent. It helps prevent build up of cholesterol on the arterial walls, thus reducing chances of strokes. Being rich in alpha-carotene, pumpkin is believed to slow the process of aging and also prevent cataract formation.

Pumpkin Scones

1 ½ cups whole wheat flour

2 cups unbleached flour

¼ cup organic cane sugar

2 Tbsp ground ginger

1 Tbsp cardamom

1 Tbsp nutmeg

2 tsp baking powder

½ tsp sea salt

2/3 cup palm shortening

15 oz canned pumpkin

1 Tbsp agave

½ cup chopped walnuts

In a large mixing bowl, combine the flours, sugar, ginger, cardamom, nutmeg, baking powder, and salt. Cut in the palm shortening.   Add pumpkin and agave. Fold in the walnuts.

On a lightly floured surface, knead dough a few times, pushing it into a large circle, a few inches thick. Place on a baking sheet and cut into wedges. Bake at 425 degrees for 12-15 minutes until golden brown. Sprinkle with confectioners' sugar after baking, or sugar crystals before baking.

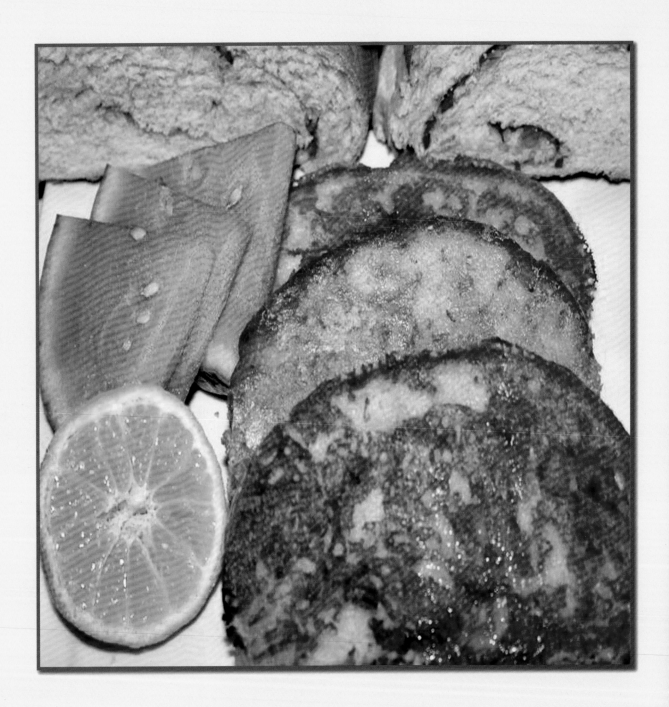

French Toast

Batter

½ cup nuts– cashews, sunflower seeds or macadamia nuts

½ cup raw oats– or substitute oats for millet, corn, quinoa

¼ cup organic cane sugar

1 Tbsp vanilla extract

¼ tsp cinnamon

dash of nutmeg, and turmeric, and paprika

sea salt

1 cup liquid– milk or water

Blend raw oats first into a powder.

Put all ingredients into a blender, processing until smooth.

For best results, use day–old bread. Pour the batter into a deep and wide dish. Dip bread slices into the batter and coat both sides. Place onto a heated non stick skillet with little or no oil, browning on both sides. Keep warm in the oven until ready to serve.

Peach, Banana Oat Muffins

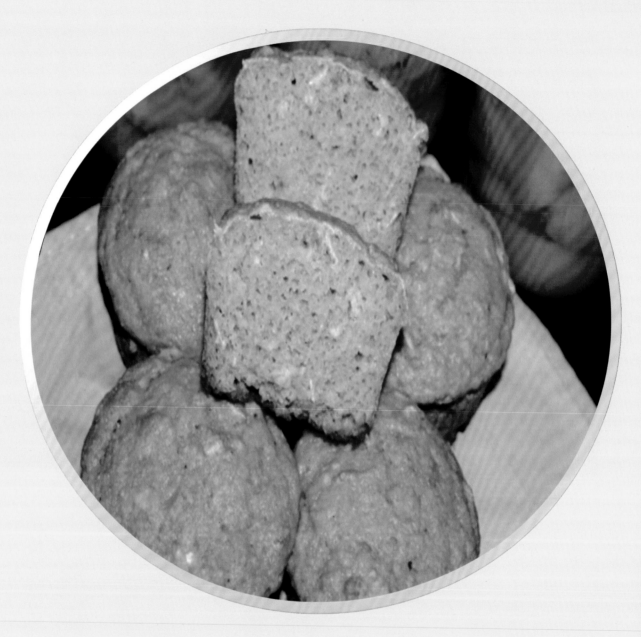

Researchers have suggested that peaches have good to excellent antioxidant activity, some antimicrobial activity and good to excellent tumor growth inhibition activity. Peaches have a small laxative effect and a powerful diuretic effect and thus, are recommended to people suffering from rheumatism and gout.

Peach, Banana Oat Muffins

1 cup unbleached all purpose flour

1 cup whole wheat flour

½ cup rolled oats

1/3 –1/2 cup organic cane sugar

1 ½ tsp baking powder

½ tsp sea salt

2 ripe bananas, mashed

2 tsp walnut oil

½ cup nut milk

1 Tbsp vanilla extract

1 cup canned peaches, drained

½ cup chopped walnuts

Preheat oven to 350 degrees.

In a mixing bowl, combine the flours, oats, sugar, baking powder and salt. In a separate bowl, combine the bananas, oil, milk, and vanilla extract. Pour the wet mixture into the flour mixture and mix well. Fold in the peaches and walnuts.

Pour batter into lined or oiled muffin pans and bake for 20–25 minutes or until toothpick inserted near center comes out clean. This recipe is not overly sweet. If more sweetness is desired, just add some of the liquid from peaches while reducing the amount of milk evenly instead of adding more sugar.

Fresh Fruit Muesli Rolls

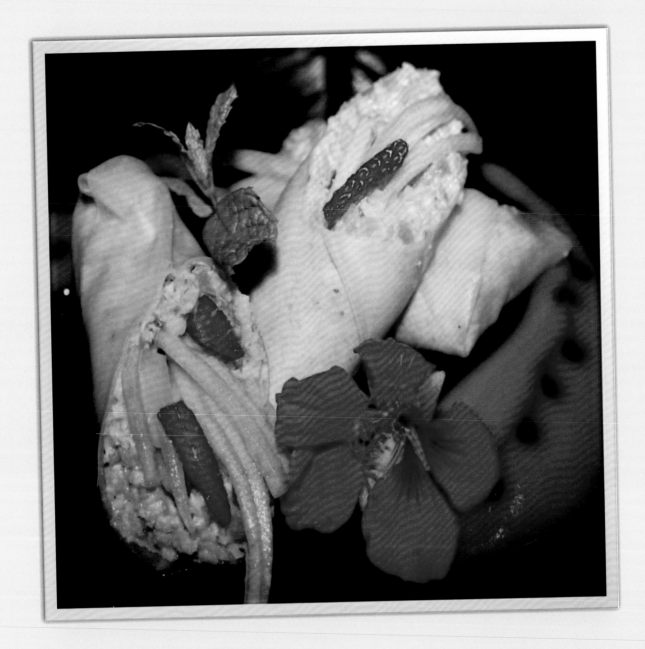

The original recipe also advised soaking the oats in water overnight as raw oats need a lengthy soaking to soften them before eating. This long soaking time is unnecessary with modern rolled "quick oats", which the manufacturers have already softened through a steam treatment.

Fresh Fruit Muesli Rolls

½ cup chopped macadamia nuts or almonds

1 cup rolled wheat

1 cup rolled rye flakes

1 cup shredded or flaked coconut

¼ cup coconut milk

¼ cup pineapple juice

½ cup orange juice

1 cup medium or thick rolled oats

½ cup dried papaya

½ cup dried pineapple

¼ cup wheat germ

¼ cup golden raisins

fresh fruit of your choice

round rice paper for summer rolls

In a food processor, cut the nuts and dried fruits into pieces about pea size. Mix together store in an airtight container until ready for use.

Combine the oats, wheat, rye flakes and coconut. This may also be stored in an airtight container for later use. Mix the coconut milk, pineapple juice and orange juice. Add ½ cup of the grain mixture (called Muesli) in the coconut milk and juices mixture and soak overnight.

When ready to roll, soak a sheet of rice paper in a shallow container filled with hot water. Allow to soften for a minute until it becomes transparent. Remove from the water and allow excess water to drip off. Place the rice paper on a flat surface and spoon a portion of the Muesli in the middle. Add a few slices of fresh fruit. Begin at the edge closest to you and fold up. Fold in the left and right edges. Then roll from the bottom towards the open top, tucking in as you roll. Repeat with remaining sheets, filling and fruit.

To serve: slice rolls in half and lay on a serving dish. Garnish with more fruit pieces and drizzle with maple or agave syrup, and/or fruit puree. Tuck in a sprig of mint, if desired.

Potato Pancake

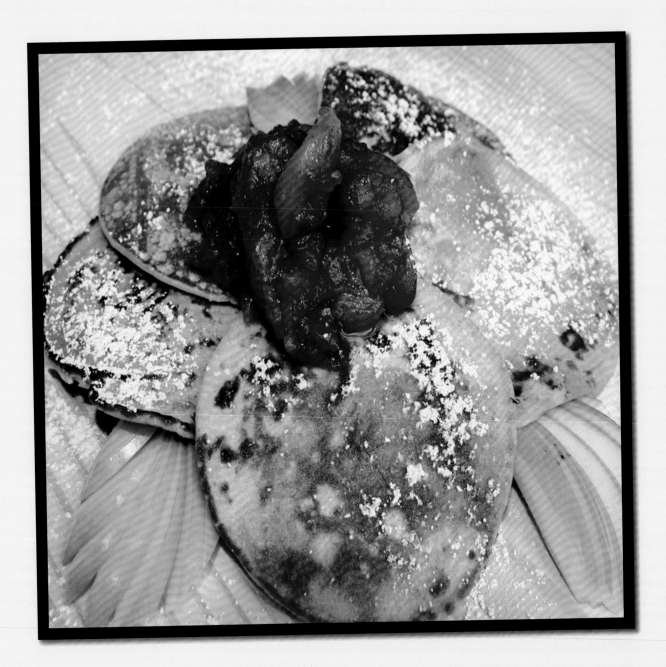

Potato Pancake

1 cup millet flour

1/3 cup sorghum flour

1/3 cup fine corn meal

1 tsp cinnamon

1 tsp nutmeg

1 tsp baking powder

¼ tsp xanthan gum

¼ tsp sea salt

1 ½ cups potatoes, peeled and diced

1 ½ cups water

2/3 cup milk

1 Tbsp vanilla extract

Olive oil for cooking

In a medium bowl, mix the flours, cornmeal, cinnamon, nutmeg, baking powder, xanthan gum and sea salt, set aside. In a blender, add the potatoes with the water and process until smooth. Add the milk and vanilla extract to the blender and mix. Pour this mixture into the dry ingredients and stir well to combine. Heat a non-stick skillet with a few drops of oil over medium-high heat. Ladle 3 ounces of batter at a time and wait till bubbles form and edges are dry. Flip over and cook until golden brown. Place on a heat-proof dish and keep in a warm oven until ready to serve.

Apple Topping

2 large apples peeled, cored and sliced

2 Tbsp agave or other sweetener

¼ organic apple juice

1 Tbsp cornstarch mixed with 2 Tbsp water

½ tsp cinnamon

¼ tsp vanilla extract

Pinch of sea salt

In a saucepan, heat apples over medium heat. Stir often until they soften. Add the apple juice, sweetener, salt and cinnamon. Cover with a lid and cook until apples are completely softened. Add vanilla and the cornstarch mixture, continuing to cook until thickened. Serve over potato pancakes.

Cornmeal Waffles

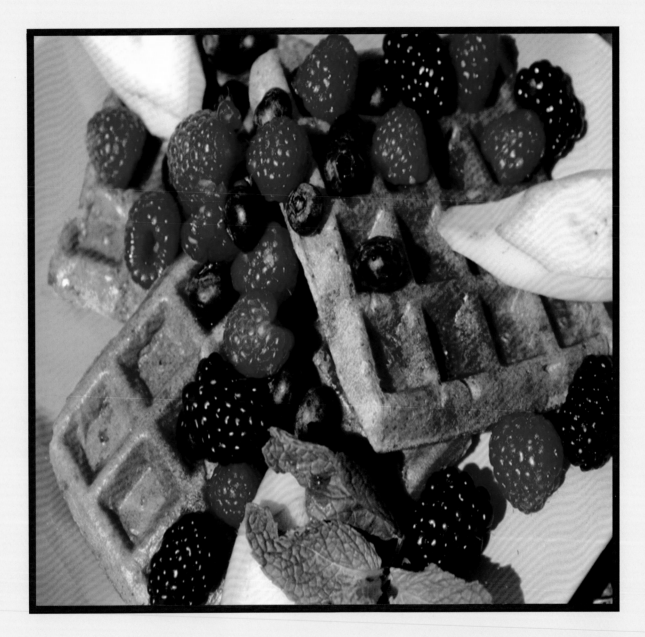

These are great and hearty waffles, topped with fresh fruit or even a fruit soup. Is a nice start for the day, or light supper for the evening.

Cornmeal Waffles

1 cup cooked cornmeal

10 dates

½ cup sunflower seeds

1 tsp sea salt

3 cups water

1 cup whole wheat flour

2 cups rolled oats

½ tsp cardamom

1 tsp coriander

¼ cup flax meal

In a blender, add the cornmeal, dates, sunflower seeds, sea salt and half the water. Blend until liquefied. Add in the remaining water with the flour, oats, cardamom, coriander and flax meal. Blend until just combined. Heat the waffle iron while letting the batter sit. Once it is heated, pour in the batter. Cooking time depends on your waffle iron.

Peanut Butter Cookies

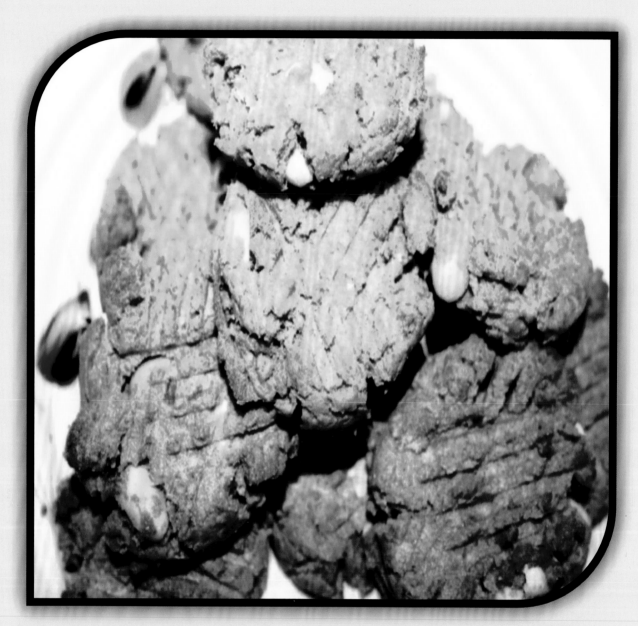

Yacon root is considered the world's richest source of fructooligosaccharide (FOS), a unique type of sugar that can't be absorbed by the body. FOS acts as a prebiotic, serving as food for the "friendly" bacteria in the colon, and preclinical studies have indicated that consumption of FOS may help increase bone density and protect against osteoporosis.

Peanut Butter Cookies

1 cup whole wheat flour

½ tsp baking powder

4 Tbsp palm shortening

2 Tbsp yacon syrup

2Tbsp apple sauce

½ cup maple syrup

½ cup peanut butter

1 Tbsp molasses

1 Tbsp vanilla

¼ cup peanut halves

¼ tsp salt

Preheat oven to 325 degrees F.

In a mixing bowl, stir together flour, baking powder and salt.

In a second bowl, shortening, yacon and maple syrup, vanilla, apple sauce, peanut butter, peanuts. Stir until smooth.

Add flour mixture to apple mixture and stir until mixed. Form dough into 16 equal pieces and shape pieces into balls. Press down slightly to make neat mounds. Place the 16 mounds about 2 1/2 inches apart on an ungreased cookie sheet and use a fork and press a criss-cross pattern on top of each cookie. These don't spread much, so if you don't press the criss-cross, make sure you shape the cookies neatly.

Bake for 15 minutes. Let cool for 3 minute on sheet, then transfer to wire rack to cool.

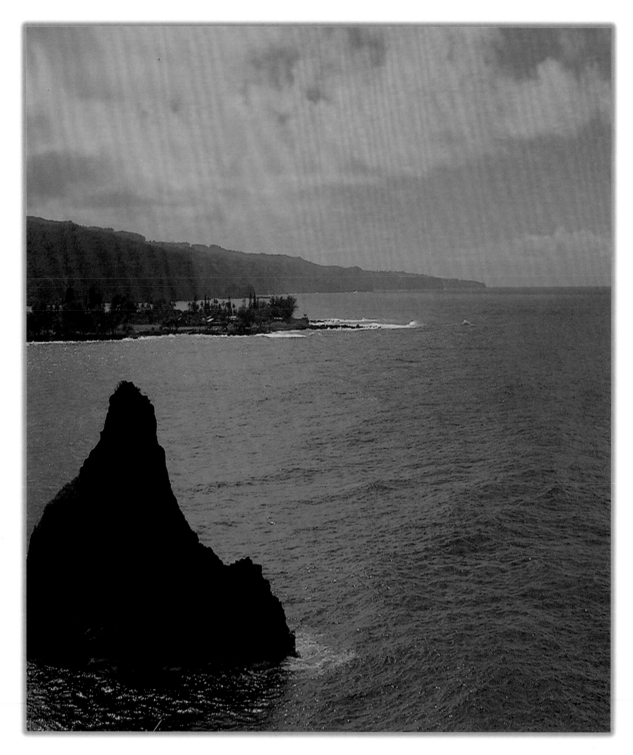

From the east shore of Maui rugged cliffs we can catch a glimpse of Keanea peninsula. This area is a bird sanctuary called "Bird Island" by the locals that live there. This private spot can only be accessed by taking a one mile hike through the lush Keanea jungle.

White Sauce

½ cup cashews

¼ tsp salt

½ cup oil

½ cup water

1 tsp yellow mustard

2 –3 clove garlic

2 Tbsp lemon juice

1 tsp soy sauce

In a blender, combine all ingredients except oil and blend till smooth. While blending on high, pour the oil in slowly, and adjust flavors as needed. To this white sauce base, you can add other flavors to make different sauces. Try these: Pesto, Chinese black beans (fermented soybeans, also called Douchi), Chipotle, Curry powder, Pepper pods, Fresh Herbs.

Teriyaki Sauce

1 Tbsp. sesame oil

1 large ginger root, pounded

1 whole bulb of garlic, pounded

½ cup soy sauce

1½ cup water

¾ cup organic cane sugar

1 whole lemon

1 Tbsp. crushed red pepper

cornstarch, to thicken

Heat oil in a saucepan; add ginger and garlic, sauté until softened. Add remaining ingredients except cornstarch, and bring to a boil, stirring occasionally. Reduce heat to low and simmer for 15 minutes. Adjust taste as necessary. Strain out liquid, discarding the solids, and replace to the saucepan. Using a whisk, add the cornstarch mixture and bring to a boil to thicken. Remove from heat and use immediately or store in refrigerator up to one week.

Indian Curry Powder

1 part cumin	1 part paprika	1 part curry powder
1 part turmeric	1 part onion powder	1 part garlic powder
1 part fennel powder	1 part ground oregano	1 part coriander
½ part cinnamon	½ part nutmeg	¼ part ground cloves

Adding Garam Masala to this mixture would make it taste quite authentic.

Combine all ingredients with 2 parts salt - use either a spoon measure or cup measure. Store in a dry place.

Suggested uses

For breads- use olive oil fresh cilantro.

Oven roasted potatoes- add olive oil and freshly chopped garlic.

For sauce- add seasonings to coconut milk, and thicken with cornstarch, sea salt.

Curry mayo- add to your favorite type of vegan mayonnaise.

Add to our white sauce to flavor any dish with.

For soups and stews.

Marinara Sauce

2 Tbsp olive oil

½ medium onion, small diced

½ green bell pepper small dice

3 cloves garlic, chopped

½ tsp fresh thyme

1 Tbsp fresh parsley

1 tsp fresh basil

sea salt to taste

3 ½ cups whole, peeled, canned tomatoes in puree (about 1 (28-ounce) can), or fresh

Heat the oil in a medium saucepan over medium-high heat. Add the onion, bell pepper and garlic, and cook stirring, until lightly browned, about 3 minutes. Add the tomatoes, their juice, and bring to a boil. Adjust the heat to maintain a simmer, and cook covered, for 10 minutes. Add the herbs and chopped fresh tomatoes, if using, and simmer for a few more minutes until fresh tomatoes are cooked through.   Stir in the salt, to taste.

Garam Masala

4 Tbsp coriander seeds

1 Tbsp cumin seed

1 ½ Tbsp dry ginger

1 ½ Tbsp black cumin seeds

¾ tsp black cardamom (3-4 large pods approx)

¾ tsp cloves

¾ tsp cinnamon (2 X 1" pieces)

¾ tsp crushed bay leaves

Heat a heavy skillet on a medium flame and gently roast all ingredients (leave cardamom in its pods till later) except the dry ginger, till they turn a few shades darker. Stir occasionally. Do not be tempted to speed up the process by turning up the heat as the spices will burn on the outside and remain raw on the inside.

When the spices are roasted turn of the flame and allow them to cool. Once cooled, remove the cardamom seeds from their skins and mix them back with all the other roasted spices.

Grind them all together, to a fine powder in a clean, dry coffee grinder. Store in a dry place.

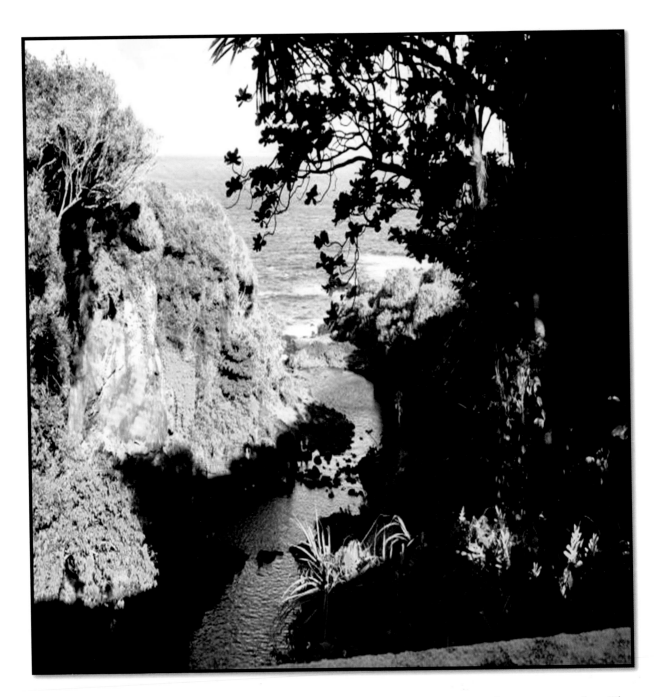

This series of tranquil pools trails through the O'heo Gulch flows into the ocean nearby. The Pipiwai Streams feeds these falls and numerous pool starting 2 miles inland. But the easiest to reach and the nicest pools are located near the shoreline. The other famous name given to this spot is called the Seven Sacred Pools of Kipahulu, even though there are more than seven.

Home Remedies

This section has been compiled for times when a doctor or physician cannot be reached. This is information that I have gathered through the years, talking with people that work in the field of health and preventative medicines. These are only **suggestions** you could use or maybe already do use. Please feel free to do more research about these products; the more closely the healing agent is to nature, the more able the body will be able to respond to it. I myself take no pharmaceutical products- and am always eager to do any "new" methods of healing and cleansing I have learned about. Remember to use only certified organic products and filtered water when doing any type of remedies. Natural remedies will tend to have better results when not mixed with other conventional, pharmaceutical, drugs.

Activated charcoal is as an emergency decontaminant in the gastrointestinal tract, which includes the stomach and intestines. Activated charcoal is considered to be the most effective single agent available. It is used after a person swallows or absorbs almost any toxic drug or chemical. From bee stings, centipedes, snake bites to cyanide poising, from rashes to the flu one of the first things we go for in our home is charcoal. We also use it for animals as well with same outstanding results.

Cayenne pepper actually can raise the body temperature a bit, as it stimulates circulation and blood flow to the skin. An herb such as cayenne or ginger that promotes fever and sweating is considered to have a diaphoretic (sweat-inducing) action. This action can help reduce fevers and relieve such the congestion of colds and sinusitis. Cayenne has become a popular home treatment for mild high blood pressure and high blood cholesterol levels. Cayenne preparations prevent platelets from clumping together and accumulating in the blood, allowing the blood to flow more easily. Since it is thought to help improve circulation, it's often used by those who have cold hands and feet. In the case of children with fevers, the best way i have seen it done (to my child). Is to get a stock pot of bucket big enough to put their feet inside. Fill warm water to cover their feet and put 2 heaping table spoon of cayenne into it, then place their feet in the water for about 5- 10 minutes and the fever should go away, with no discomfort to the child.

Chia Seed For centuries this tiny little seed was used as a staple food by the Indians of the south west and Mexico. Known as the running food, its use as a high energy endurance food has been recorded as far back as the ancient Aztecs. It was said the Aztec warriors subsisted on the Chia seed during the conquests. 30% of chia seed oil is Omega 3 oil. 10% of its oil is Omega 6 oil. This is the perfect balance of essential fatty acids. Studies show that eating chia seed slows down how fast our bodies convert carbohydrate calories into simple sugars. This leads scientists to believe that the chia seed may have great benefits for diabetics. The chia seed gels when becoming wet and this gel, when in our digestive systems, helps prevent some of the food, hence calories that we eat from getting absorbed into our system. This blockage of calorie absorption makes the chia seed a great diet helper. Eating the seeds also helps dieters by making them feel fuller faster so they will be less hungry.

Coffee Enema this cleans the liver of all its toxins. Used by many professionals in the natural treatment of cancer. I will not list the procedure but you can find out more about on the web

Colloidal Silver As an alternative antibiotic, is known to kill most germs - viruses, fungi, bacteria and internal parasites - Fighting viral infections, colds, flu, yeast and fungal infections without side effects or harm to humans, animals or plants, and also promotes wound healing and tissue growth. This is another super product that is safe and proven time and time again. The closer you can get the product to the area, the faster you will see results. It cannot be beat or topical cuts and wounds, and the product is also sterile, so you could use it as a sanitizer. We have a great contact that has one of the best silver on the market, and the work that they are doing is mind blowing.

Flax Seed Some call it one of the most powerful plant foods on the planet. There's some evidence it can help reduce your risk of heart disease, cancer, stroke, and diabetes. Omega-3 fatty acids are a key force against inflammation in our bodies. Mounting evidence shows that inflammation plays a part in many chronic diseases including heart disease, arthritis, asthma, diabetes, and even some cancers. This inflammation is enhanced by having too little Omega-3 intake (such as in fish, flax, and walnuts), especially in relation to Omega-6 fatty acid intake (in such oils as soy and corn oil). In the quest to equalize the ratio of these two kinds of oils, flax seed can be a real help. Flax seeds are also beneficial for making poultices in which it draws out toxins from the body.

Gall Bladder Cleanse There is a lot of information on the internet about this cleanse, using organic apple juice, Epsom salt, lemon and olive oil.

Grapefruit Seed Extract Grapefruit seed extract is being used successfully in humans and animals alike to eliminate many types of internal and external infections caused from many types of parasites (single and multi-celled), viruses, bacteria's, funguses and more! It naturally detoxifies, enhances and supports the immune system. It has been proven highly effective in numerous applications. Physicians have observed that the herpes simplex virus becomes inactive just ten minutes after the application of grapefruit seed extract. Grapefruit seed extract contains high levels of vitamin C and E, and bioflavonoid. The important substances have an antioxidant action and can neutralize free radicals that damage cells and cause a number of illnesses. Grapefruit seed extract is nontoxic. Because grapefruit seed extract is non toxic and does not exhibit the harsh side effects and high cost of pharmaceuticals it is becoming the alternative health choice for naturopathic physicians, clinics and the general public. We would use it anytime we want kill any flu type symptoms and safe to use on animals.

Green Juice a combination of green leafy vegetables juiced together to make a nuclear energy for the body. Kale, Swiss Chards, Collard Greens are at the top of my choices. Originally is part of cleansing program, with one part green and three parts water. This combination has more energy than any sports bar on the market today. All a person would need is 8oz of pure green juice, and rocket shoes.

Lung Tea fresh herbs, parsley, oregano, sage, thyme, when this is brewed in 3 cups of water for 15 minutes and it helps relieve some lung problems like emphysema.

Pain Relief topical Arnica cream works wonders, for minor cramps, bumps, and muscle pain. For internal pain, turmeric is a good thing to have on hand. If the pain is extreme use turmeric with vitamin c- (with blast) and stinging nettle, there is about 20 minutes of rashy skin sensation from the vitamin c blast. I would not suggest doing this at work, for they will send you home when you start looking like a lobster.

Rheumatoid Arthritis I have heard many people have been blessed by taking Royal Jelly as part of their diet. Royal Jelly is food only for the queen bees.

Rosemary Tea this tea is for times when staying awake or alert is a must- take fresh rosemary branches and make tea, strain drink cool or hot--- **Be Advised-** it is very powerful caffeine.

Wheat Grass Increases red blood-cell count and lowers blood pressure. It cleanses the blood, organs and gastrointestinal tract of debris. Wheatgrass also stimulates metabolism and the body's enzyme systems by enriching the blood. It also aids in reducing blood pressure by dilating the blood pathways throughout the body. Stimulates the thyroid gland, correcting obesity, indigestion, and a host of other complaints. Restores alkalinity to the blood. The juice's abundance of alkaline minerals helps reduce over-acidity in the blood. It can be used to relieve many internal pains, and has been used successfully to treat peptic ulcers, ulcerative colitis, constipation, diarrhea, and other complaints of the gastrointestinal tract. Is a powerful detoxifier, and liver and blood protector. The enzymes and amino acids found in wheatgrass can protect us from carcinogens like no other food or medicine. It strengthens our cells, detoxifies the liver and bloodstream, and chemically neutralizes environmental pollutants. Fights tumors and neutralizes toxins. Recent studies show that wheatgrass juice has a powerful ability to fight tumors without the usual toxicity of drugs that also inhibit cell-destroying agents. The many active compounds found in grass juice cleanse the blood and neutralize and digest toxins in our cells. Contains beneficial enzymes. Whether you have a cut finger you want to heal or you desire to lose five pounds...enzymes must do the actual work. The life and abilities of the enzymes found naturally in our bodies can be extended if we help them from the outside by adding exogenous enzymes, like the ones found in wheatgrass juice. Don't cook it. We can only get the benefits of the many enzymes found in grass by eating it uncooked. Cooking destroys 100 percent of the enzymes in food. I have used only the fresh product which grew on the slopes of Maui, in the fertile earth. When I did use it, I had nothing but positive results. Information I got from the grower was, the roots need the ground to release the sugar in the grass, if they are planted in trays, the sugar content is too high, and not good for diabetics.

If you would like more information please feel free to contact us through our web site.

www.TheMauiVegetarian.com

The Impending Conflict

Satan's power to deceive can be very great—when men choose to remain ignorant. In every age there has been a decided struggle of truth against error. But the greatest one is just ahead. One of the most massive crises of the ages is just before mankind. Of Babylon at this time, it is declared in Scripture, "Her sins have reached unto Heaven, and God hath remembered her iniquities." Revelation 13 predicts that a time is just before us when those who honor fundamental Bible truths will be denounced as enemies of law and order. We must individually know the Word of God for ourselves, that we may stand on the right side in that day —

And he doeth great wonders, so that he maketh fire come down from heaven on the earth in the sight of men, And deceiveth them that dwell on the earth by the means of those miracles which he had power to do in the sight of the beast; saying to them that dwell on the earth, that they should make an image to the beast, which had the wound by a sword, and did live. And he had power to give life unto the image of the beast. That the image of the beast should both speak, and cause that as many as would not worship the image of the beast should be killed. **And he causeth all, both small and great, rich and poor, free and bond, to receive a mark in their right hand, or in their foreheads:** And that no man might buy or sell, save he that had the mark, or the name of the beast, or the number of his name.

"Satan is exercising his power. He sweeps away the ripening harvest, and famine and distress follow. He imparts to the air a deadly taint, and thousands perish by the pestilence. These visitations are to become more and more frequent and disastrous."—
EGW, Great Controversy, 590.

"On one occasion, when in New York City, I was in the night season called upon to behold buildings rising story after story toward heaven . . The scene that next passed before me was an alarm of fire. Men looked at the lofty and supposedly fireproof buildings and said: 'They are perfectly safe.' But these buildings were consumed as if made of pitch. The fire engines could do nothing to stay the destruction. The firemen were unable to operate the engines."—*EGW, 9 Testimonies, 12-13 (1909).*

"In the night I was, I thought, in a room but not in my own house. I was in a city, where I knew not, and I heard explosion after explosion. I rose up quickly in bed, and saw from my window large balls of fire. Jetting out were sparks, in the form of arrows, and buildings were being consumed, and in a very few minutes the entire block of buildings was falling and the screeching and mournful groans came distinctly to my ears. I cried out, in my raised position, to learn what was happening: Where am I? And where are our family circle? Then I awoke." —*EGW, Manuscript126 (1906).*

"During a vision of the night, I stood on an eminence, from which I could see houses shaken like a reed in the wind. Buildings, great and small, were falling to the ground. Pleasure resorts, theaters, hotels, and the homes of the wealthy were shaken and shattered. Many lives were blotted out of existence, and the air was filled with the shrieks of the injured and the terrified . . One touch, and buildings, so thoroughly constructed that men regarded them as secure against every danger, quickly became heaps of rubbish. There was no assurance of safety in any place."—*EGW, 9 Testimonies, 92-93 (1909).*

"The crisis is stealing gradually upon us. The sun shines in the heavens, passing over its usual round, and the heavens still declare the glory of God. Men are still eating and drinking, planting and building, marrying and giving in marriage. Merchants are still buying and selling. Men are jostling one against another, contending for the highest place. Pleasure lovers are still crowding to theaters, horse races, gambling hells. The highest excitement prevails, yet probation's hour is fast closing, and every case is about to be eternally decided. Satan sees that his time is short. He has set all his agencies at work that men may be deceived, deluded, occupied, and entranced until the day of probation shall be ended, and the door of mercy forever shut."—*EGW, Southern Watchman, Oct. 3, 1905.*

As spiritualism more closely imitates the nominal Christianity of the day, it has greater power to deceive andensnare. Satan himself is converted after the modern order of things. He will appear in the character of an angel of light. Through the agency of spiritualism, miracles will be wrought, the sick will be healed, and many undeniable wonders will be performed. And as the spirits will profess faith in the Bible and manifest respect for the institutions of the church, their work will be accepted as a manifestation ofdivine power.

Through spiritualism, Satan appears as a benefactor of the race, healing the diseases of the people, and professing to present a new and more exalted system of religious faith; but at the same time he works as a destroyer. His temptations are leading multitudes to ruin. Intemperance dethrones reason; sensual indulgence, strife, and bloodshed follow.

Fearful is the issue to which the world is to be brought. The powers of earth, uniting to war against the commandments of God, will decree that all, "both small and great, rich and poor, free and bond" (Rev. 13:16), shall conform to the customs of the church by the observance of the false sabbath. All who refuse compliance will be visited with civil penalties, and it will finally be declared that they are deserving of death. On the other hand, the law of God enjoining the Creator's rest day demands obedience, and threatens wrath against all who transgress its precepts. With the issue thus clearly brought before him, whoever shall trample upon God's law to obey a human enactment, receives the mark of the beast; he accepts the sign of allegiance to the power which he chooses to obey instead of God. The warning from Heaven is, "If any man worship the beast and his image, and receive his mark in his forehead, or in his hand, the same shall drink of the wine of the wrath of God, which is poured out without mixture into the cup of His indignation.

A Call to Leave the Cities

The Perils of the Cities

Few realize the importance of shunning, so far as possible, all associations unfriendly to religious life. In choosing their surroundings, few make their spiritual prosperity the first consideration.

Parents flock with their families to the cities, because they fancy it easier to obtain a livelihood there than in the country. The children, having nothing to do when not in school, obtain a street education. From evil associates, they acquire habits of vice and dissipation. The parents see all this, but it will require a sacrifice to correct their error, and they stay where they are, until Satan gains full control of their children.

Better sacrifice any and every worldly consideration than to imperil the precious souls committed to your care. They will be assailed by temptations, and should be taught to meet them; but it is your duty to cut off every influence, to break up every habit, to sunder every tie, that keeps you from the most free, open, and hearty committal of yourselves and your family to God.

Instead of the crowded city, seek some retired situation where your children will be, so far as possible, shielded from temptation, and there train and educate them for usefulness. The prophet Ezekiel thus enumerates the causes that led to Sodom's sin and destruction: "Pride, fullness of bread, and abundance of idleness was in her and in her daughters; neither did she strengthen the hands of the poor and needy." All who would escape the doom of Sodom, must shun the course that brought God's judgments upon that wicked city.-- Testimonies, vol. 5, pp. 232, 233. (1882)

City Living Not God's Plan

The world over, cities are becoming hotbeds of vice. On every hand are the sights and sounds of evil. Everywhere are enticements to sensuality and dissipation. The tide of corruption and crime is continually swelling. Every day brings the record of violence, --robberies, murders, suicides, and crimes unnamable.

Life in the cities is false and artificial. The intense passion for money getting, the whirl of excitement and pleasure seeking, the thirst for display, the luxury and extravagance, all are forces that, with the great masses of mankind, are turning the mind from life's true purpose. They are opening the door to a thousand evils. Upon the youth they have almost irresistible power.

One of the most subtle and dangerous temptations that assails the children and youth in the cities is the love of pleasure. Holidays are numerous; games and horse racing draw thousands, and the whirl of excitement and pleasure attracts them away from the sober duties of life. Money that should have been saved for better uses is frittered away for amusements.

Through the working of trusts, and the results of labor unions and strikes the conditions of life in the city are constantly becoming more and more difficult. Serious troubles are before us; and for many families removal from the cities will become a necessity.

The physical surroundings in the cities are often a peril to health. The constant liability to contact with disease, the prevalence of foul air, impure water, impure food, the crowded, dark, unhealthful dwellings, are some of the many evils to be met.

It was not God's purpose that people should be crowded into cities, huddled together in terraces and tenements. In the beginning He placed our first parents amidst the beautiful sights and sounds He desires us to rejoice in today. The more nearly we come into harmony with God's original plan, the more favorable will be our position to secure health of body, and mind, and soul.--The Ministry of Healing, pp. 363-365. (1905)

A Loitering Spirit

I could not sleep past two o'clock this morning. During the night season I was in council. I was pleading with some families to avail themselves of God's appointed means, and get away from the cities to save their children. Some were loitering, making no determined efforts.

The angels of mercy hurried Lot and his wife and daughters by taking hold of their hands. Had Lot hastened as the Lord desired him to, his wife would not have become a pillar of salt. Lot had too much of a lingering spirit. Let us not be like him. The same voice that warned Lot to leave Sodom bids us, "Come out from among them, and be ye separate, . . . and touch not the unclean." Those who obey this warning will find a refuge. Let every man be wide awake for himself, and try to save his family. Let him gird himself for the work. God will reveal from point to point what to do next.

Hear the voice of God through the apostle Paul: "Work out your own salvation with fear and trembling. For it is God which worketh in you both to will and to do of His good pleasure." Lot trod the plain with unwilling and tardy steps. He had so long associated with evil workers that he could not see his peril until his wife stood on the plain a pillar of salt forever.--Review and Herald, Dec. 11, 1900.

Cities to Be Visited by God's Judgments

The time is near when the large cities will be visited by the judgments of God. In a little while, these cities will be terribly shaken. No matter how large or how strong their buildings, no matter how many safeguards against fire may have been provided, let God touch these buildings, and in a few minutes or a few hours they are in ruins.

The ungodly cities of our world are to be swept away by the besom of destruction. In the calamities that are now befalling immense buildings and large portions of cities, God is showing us what will come upon the whole earth.--Testimonies, vol. 7, pp. 82, 83. (1902)

Results of Unheeded Warnings

I am bidden to declare the message that cities full of transgression, and sinful in the extreme, will be destroyed by earthquakes, by fire, by flood. All the world will be warned that there is a God who will display His authority as God. His unseen agencies will cause destruction, devastation, and death. All the accumulated riches will be as nothingness. . . .

Calamities will come--calamities most awful, most unexpected; and these destructions will follow one after another. If there will be a heeding of the warnings that God has given, and if churches will repent, returning to their allegiance, then other cities may be spared for a time. But if men who have been deceived continue in the same way in which they have been walking, disregarding the law of God, and presenting falsehoods before the people, God allows them to suffer calamity, that their senses may be awakened.

The Lord will not suddenly cast off all transgressors, or destroy entire nations; but He will punish cities and places where men have given themselves up to the possession of Satanic agencies. Strictly will the cities of the nations be dealt with, and yet they will not be visited in the extreme of God's indignation, because some souls will yet break away from the delusions of the enemy, and will repent and be converted, while the mass will be treasuring up wrath against the day of wrath.--Evangelism, p. 27. (1906)

Imminence of God's Judgments

There are reasons why we should not build in the cities. On these cities, God's judgments are soon to fall.--Letter 158, 1902.

The time is near when large cities will be swept away, and all should be warned of these coming judgments.--Evangelism, p. 29. (1910)

O that God's people had a sense of the impending destruction of thousands of cities, now almost given to idolatry.--Review and Herald, Sept. 10, 1903.

A View of Great Destruction

Last Friday morning, just before I awoke, a very impressive scene was presented before me. I seemed to awake from sleep, but was not in my home. From the windows I could behold a terrible conflagration. Great balls of fire were falling upon houses, and from these balls fiery arrows were flying in every direction. It was impossible to check the fires that were kindled, and many places were being destroyed. The terror of the people was indescribable. --Evangelism, p. 29. (1906)

God's Efforts to Arouse the People

While at Loma Linda, Calif., April 16, 1906, there passed before me a most wonderful representation. During a vision of the night, I stood on an eminence, from which I could see houses shaken like a reed in the wind. Buildings, great and small, were falling to the ground. Pleasure resorts, theaters, hotels, and the homes of the wealthy were shaken and shattered. Many lives were blotted out of existence, and the air was filled with the shrieks of the injured and the terrified.

The destroying angels of God were at work. One touch, and buildings so thoroughly constructed that men regarded them as secure against every danger, quickly became heaps of rubbish. There was no assurance of safety in any place. I did not feel in any special peril, but the awfulness of the scenes that passed before me I cannot find words to describe. It seemed that the forbearance of God was exhausted, and that the judgment day had come.

The angel that stood at my side then instructed me that but few have any conception of the wickedness existing in our world today, and especially the wickedness in the large cities. He declared that the Lord has appointed a time when He will visit transgressors in wrath for persistent disregard of His law.

Terrible as was the representation that passed before me, that which impressed itself most vividly upon my mind was the instruction given in connection with it. The angel that stood by my side declared that God's supreme rulership, and the sacredness of His law, must be revealed to those who persistently refuse to render obedience to the King of kings. Those who choose to remain disloyal, must be visited in mercy with judgments, in order that, if possible, they may be aroused to a realization of the sinfulness of their course.-- Testimonies, vol. 9, pp. 92, 93. (1909)

Peril to Those Who Remain Unnecessarily

In harmony with the light given me, I am urging people to come out from the great centers of population. Our cities are increasing in wickedness, and it is becoming more and more evident that those who remain in them unnecessarily do so at the peril of their soul's salvation.--Manuscript 115, 1907.

The following have been taken from the following books "The Great Controversy" and" Country Living" both these book were written by Ellen G.White over 100 years ago.

Then shall the dust return to the earth as it was: and the spirit shall return unto God who gave it. Vanity of vanities, saith the preacher; all [is] vanity. And moreover, because the preacher was wise, he still taught the people knowledge; yea, he gave good heed, and sought out, [and] set in order many proverbs. The preacher sought to find out acceptable words: and [that which was] written [was] upright, [even] words of truth. The words of the wise [are] as goads, and as nails fastened [by] the masters of assemblies, [which] are given from one shepherd. And further, by these, my son, be admonished: of making many books [there is] no end; and much study [is] a weariness of the flesh.   Let us hear the conclusion of the whole matter. Fear God, and keep his commandments: for this [is] the whole [duty] of man. For God shall bring every work into judgment, with every secret thing, whether [it be] good, or whether [it be] evil.

My hope and prayer for myself and the reader is that we can stand in our lot before the God of the universe when he comes and say that we truly know him. May you be blessed by this counsel and take the proper precautions to weather the coming storm. Noah was thought to be a lunatic, a crazy man. History shows he and his family were the only ones separated from the world; they didn't need a crash course on swimming. Even though I am a certified rescue diver, I cannot save myself from this storm, only Messiah Yashua will be able to save any of us...reach for His arm....

Glossary

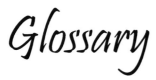

Achiote -Annato seed is also known as achiote. This seed grows on the annato tree. It is used primarily in Mexican and Caribbean cooking to impart a rich yellow/orange color. Annato seed makes a good substitute for saffron's golden coloring, at a fraction of the cost. It does NOT, however, duplicate saffron's unique flavor!

Agave-To produce agave nectar from the Agave tequiliana plant, juice is expressed from the core of the agave, called the piña. The juice is filtered, then heated to hydrolyze polysaccharides into simple sugars. The main polysaccharide is called inulin or fructosan and comprises mostly fructose units. The filtered, hydrolyzed juice is concentrated to a syrup-like liquid a little thinner than honey that ranges in color from light to dark depending on the degree of processing.

Bais- to cut at an angle

Buckwheat flour-flour ground from *Fagopyrum esculentum*, known more casually as buckwheat. It has a rich, nutty flavor and a very high nutritional value, making it popular in many nations, especially in Asia. In addition, buckwheat flour is gluten free, leading people with gluten intolerance to seek it out as a flour alternative.

Caramelize- is just cooking so they brown deeply. It's easy to do and results in cooked with a dark, sweet, browned flavor. You're really turning the sugars within the product to caramel - hence the name.

Cardamom- comes from the seeds of a ginger-like plant. The small, brown-black sticky seeds are contained in a pod in three double rows with about six seeds in each row. The pods are between 5-20 mm (1/4"-3/4") long, the larger variety known as 'black', being brown and the smaller being green. White-bleached pods are also available

Capers-are buds from the juniper berry tree- the same tree they make gin from. It's usually marinated and sold in brine.

Carob -The carob tree grows in the Mediterranean and is scientifically called Ceratonia siliqua. It is a member of the legume family and produces pods that are long and leathery. Within these pods are hard seeds and pulp. The pulp is edible and has a sweet flavor.

Corn meal—is flour ground from dried corn. It is a common staple food, and is ground to fine, medium, and coarse consistencies. In the United States, the finely ground cornmeal is also referred to as corn flour.

Dates- are oval-cylindrical, 3–7 cm long, and 2–3 cm diameter, and when unripe, range from bright red to bright yellow in color, depending on variety. The type of fruit depends on the glucose, fructose and sucrose content.

Degorge -The process of sprinkling vegetables with salt to eliminate water. Eggplant, cucumbers and cabbage are often salted, rinsed quickly and patted dry before cooking

Douchi - a traditional fermented soybean product that originated in China, has been consumed since ancient times as a food seasoning.

Egg Replacer-Mimics what eggs do in recipes, greatly simplifies baking for people who cannot use eggs. It replaces egg whites as well as egg yolks in baking.

Elephant garlic-is probably more closely related to the leek than to ordinary garlic. The bulbs are very large and can weigh over a pound. A single clove of elephant garlic can be as large as a whole bulb of ordinary garlic, is much sweeter and milder than regular garlic.

Flax oil-Flaxseed oil is derived from the seeds of the flax plant. Flaxseed oil and flaxseed contain substances that promote good health. One of these substances is alpha-linolenic acid (ALA), an essential fatty acid that appears to be beneficial for heart disease, inflammatory bowel disease, arthritis, and other health conditions.

Flax meal- Flax has a pleasantly nutty taste. The whole seeds keep well, but they need to be ground into meal for us to get their full nutritional benefit. A simple spice or coffee grinder can do this in seconds.

Garam Masala-from Hindi garam ("hot") and masala ("mixture") is a basic blend of ground spices common in Indian and other South Asian cuisines.It is used alone or with other seasonings. The word *garam* refers to spice intensity, not heat; Garam masala is pungent, but not "hot" in the same way as a chili pepper.

Garbanzo bean flour- is made from grinding Garbanzo beans (sometimes called chickpeas) to fine flour and works well by itself or blended with other bean flours

Hoisin sauce- ingredients include water, sugar, soybeans, white distilled vinegar, rice, salt, wheat flour, garlic, and red chili peppers, and several preservatives and coloring agents.

Infuse – to incorporate flavors from a product by either by heat or freezing usually in oils.

Julienne – a cutting technique in which resembles the shape of matchsticks.

Masa harina- is Spanish for dough, but in Mexico it sometimes refers to corn is Spanish for dough. It is used for making tortillas, tamales, pupusas, arepas and many other Latin American dishes. The dried and powdered form is then reconstituted with water.

 Millet- is tiny in size and round in shape and can be white, gray, yellow or red. The most widely available form of millet found in stores is the pearled, hulled variety, although traditional couscous made from cracked millet can also be found. The term millet refers to a variety of grains, some of which do not belong to the same genus.

Napa cabbage- grows in a compact, elongated head; the crinkled oblong leaves are wrapped tightly in an upright cylinder. The leaves of this cabbage are light green, and the stalk area below the leaves is lighter still, a pale green approaching white.

Nori- is the Japanese name for various edible seaweed species of the red algae, sometimes called laver. Finished products are made by a shredding and rack-drying process that resembles papermaking.

Nutritional yeast- Yellow in color and with a nutty cheesy flavor, nutritional yeast is inactive yeast that is a favorite amongst many vegans because of its unique flavor and similarity to cheese when added to foods.

New Mexico and Ancho pods-dried pepper pods of the Anaheim, Hatch" or "Mesilla Valley.

Palm shortening- Palm shortening is derived from palm oil. In its natural state, palm oil is a mixture of saturated and unsaturated fatty acids, with most of the unsaturated fat being monounsaturated fat. Palm shortening is palm oil that has some of its unsaturated fats removed, giving it a very firm texture, and high melting point.

Plum sauce-sweet sauce prepared with using plum fruits and various asian flavors.

Portabella- They are actually mature Criminis and have a meatier flavor, the result of a somewhat longer growing period. The stems are firmer in texture but can be trimmed and cooked along with the caps. Freshly harvested portabella caps are light tan, rounded and slightly rough-textured, with somewhat uneven edges and visible gills on the underside

Porcini - look the way a mushroom should: A corpulent firm white stalk and a broad dark brown cap -- if you're out walking in a European forest and come across a clump under a chestnut tree, where they're often found, you may well think you've stumbled into a fairy tale and look about for gnomes.

Raw Tahini- is handcrafted from fresh (not roasted) mechanically hulled sesame seeds, and is made using a low-temperature process (below 115 F) that preserves all of the nutrients that naturally occur in sesame seeds.

Rice vermicelli - are thin noodles made from rice, sometimes also known as rice noodles or rice sticks. They should not be confused with cellophane no are thin noodles made from rice.

Roasted red pepper- red bell peppers which have been fire roasted to remove thin layer of outside skin.

Saffron - the deep orange-colored stigmas of a type of crocus, sometimes ground to a powder.

Sambal Oelek - is made of chilies with no other additives such as garlic or spices for a simpler taste. Use this sauce to add heat to a dish without altering the other delicate flavors.

Sauté - to cook food quickly and lightly in a little oil, or fat.

Sesame oil- Expressed from sesame seed, sesame oil comes in two basic types. One is light in color and flavor and has a deliciously nutty nuance. It's excellent for everything from salad dressings to sautéing. The darker, Asian sesame oil has a much stronger flavor and fragrance and is used as a flavor accent for some Asian dishes.

Sesame tahini- is a paste made of ground sesame seeds which is used in many Near and Far East recipes

Shiitake- An edible eastern Asian mushroom having an aromatic, fleshy, golden or dark brown to blackish cap. Also called Chinese forest mushroom, golden oak mushroom, Oriental black mushroom, Emperors Mushroom.

Sorghum flour- Sorghum Flour, a millet-like grain, is America's third leading cereal crop. It is a powerhouse of nutrition and adds a superb flavor to gluten-free baking.

Spelt flour- is similar to wheat in appearance. However, spelt has a tougher husk than wheat, which may help protect the nutrients in spelt. Spelt flour has a somewhat nuttier and slightly sweeter flavor than whole wheat flour. Spelt contains more protein than wheat, and the protein in spelt is easier to digest.

Star anise- Star anise comes by its name honestly, with its star shape and a licorice taste similar to regular anise, only stronger. Star anise is the seed pod of an evergreen tree grown in southwestern China and Japan. It is about one inch high with eight segments and a dark brown rust color.

Sucanat - is non-refined cane sugar. Unlike refined and processed white sugar, Sucanat retains its molasses content; it is essentially pure dried sugar cane juice. The juice is extracted by mechanical processes, heated and cooled at which point the small brown grainy crystals are formed.

Sun dried tomato- are ripe tomatoes which are placed in the sun to remove most of the water content. Twenty pounds of fresh, ripe tomatoes will dry down to just one pound of sun dried tomatoes. Sun dried tomatoes have the same nutritional value as the fresh tomatoes they are made from.

Sushi vinegar- Japanese rice vinegar is very mild and mellow and ranges in color from colorless to pale yellow. Japanese vinegar is made from fermented rice.

Sweat- term used to in cooking out water from products, till translucent.

Sweet Thai chili sauce- Ingredients: palm sugar, red chili, vinegar, garlic, salt, water. Also see our sweet chili sauce for spring rolls. No preservatives and no artificial coloring.

Togarashi pepper- Japanese seven-spice mixture is a blend of red peppers, sansho pepper, roasted orange peel, black and white sesame seeds, seaweed, and ginger. Also known as Shichimi Togarashi.

Tamarind paste- is the pulp that surrounds the seeds of the tamarind pod. It is used in Thai cooking for making a traditional sour soup.

Quinoa- Most commonly considered a grain, quinoa is actually a relative of leafy green vegetables like spinach and Swiss chard. It is a recently rediscovered ancient "grain" once considered "the gold of the Incas."

Vanilla bean- is a flavoring derived from orchids of the genus *Vanilla* native to Mexico. Vanilla is the second most expensive spice after saffron,[ ] due to the extensive labor required to grow the vanilla seed pods. Despite the expense, it is highly valued for its flavor.

Vanilla extract- Pure vanilla extract is made with an extraction from vanilla beans in an alcoholic solution. Vanilla extract is the most common form of vanilla used today. Mexican, Tahitian, Indonesian and Bourbon vanilla are the main varieties. Bourbon vanilla is special in that it does not contain bourbon.

Vegenaise - an egg-free mayonnaise with real mayonnaise taste.

Won ton wrappers- paper thin wrapper made from wheat products, used for making Asian dumplings.

Wheat germ- The germ of a cereal is the reproductive part that germinates to grow into a plant; it is the embryo of the seed. Along with bran, germ is often a by-product of the milling that produces refined grain products.

Xanthan gum- is a microbial polysaccharide derived from the bacterium Xanthomonas campestris that is typically found in commercial salad dressings, ice creams and other suspensions or liquid products that require an emulsifier, but it can be bought for home use and is a great way to thicken and stabilize.

Yakon syrup- Yacon syrup is all-natural and vegan fruit-caramel tasting sweetener made by low temperature concentrating the juice of yacon tubers. The tubers of the yacon plant are tasty and sweet while their sugars (fructo-oligosaccharides) do not increase the blood-sugar level when digested. Therefore the syrup is safe for diabetics and suitable for reduction diets. It has prebiotic effects and has an important mineral content.

Yam noodle- Yam Noodles are fine Japanese noodles shaped like spaghetti. They are made from Devil's Tongue Yam flour (aka Konnyaku Powder) and water. They can be white or black. The white ones are semi-transparent. In Japanese. they are called "shirataki", meaning "white waterfall."

Index

Notes

Notes

Notes

Notes